Hooray
FOR
HRT

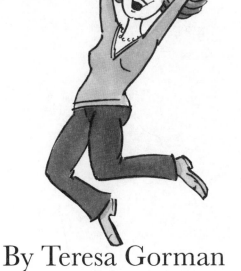

By Teresa Gorman

Published by
PAGE Publishing
3 The Capricorn Centre
Cranes Farm Road
Basildon
Essex SS14 3JA

ISBN 0-9553305-0-5

Designed by PAGE Creative Ltd
Printed by PAGE Litho Ltd
Illustrations by Bill Hopkins

ABOUT THE AUTHOR

Teresa Gorman, former teacher, scientist, businesswoman and Member of Parliament, was at the peak of her business career when, in her 40s, she began to experience the debilitating effects of the menopause.

As a result, she set up the Amarant Trust to inform other women going through the menopause of the many benefits of HRT. In doing so, she succeeded in putting HRT on the map in the UK.

Her election to Parliament in 1987 gave her the opportunity to break a taboo surrounding menopause by bringing the subject onto the floor of the House of Commons. Since then, she has contributed to menopause conferences in the UK, Sweden, Italy, Australia and Thailand.

After benefiting from thirty years on HRT, Teresa is determined that other women should not be refused HRT after five years of use because the potential damage to their health will return. In this book she attempts to set the record straight by explaining the many benefits of HRT.

ACKNOWLEDGEMENTS

I would like to thank the following for their valuable advice during the course of writing this book although they may not necessarily agree with all my views.

Professor John Studd, DSc, MD, FRCOG, Professor of Gynaecology.

Professor David W. Purdie, MD, FRCOG, FRCP Ed Consultant Osteoporosis.

Professor Nigel P.M. Sacks, MS, FRCS, FRACS, Consultant Breast & Endocrine Surgeon.

Douglas McWilliams, Chief Executive at the Centre for Economics & Business Research, for his comments on the conduct of the Million Women Study.

Dr. Amineh Abu Zayyad, for surveying current research on the genetics of breast cancer.

Fay Weldon and Wendy Cooper, for information and anecdotes.

Bill Hopkins, for his humorous illustrations.

Gillian Clarke and Maureen Koppen who researched and edited the text.

CONTENTS
"HOORAY FOR HRT"

Chapter 1

IN THE BEGINNING

Linda's letter - A Publicist's dream

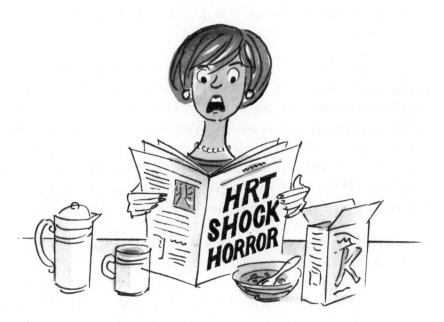

On 8th August 2003 the whole of the media was dominated by the same headline: *"HRT Doubles Risk of Breast Cancer"*. Breakfast television, radio programmes and every national newspaper landing on the doormat in millions of homes carried the same warning as a result of the publication of the Million Women Study (MWS) carried out by Cancer Research UK.

Millions of women users of hormone replacement therapy (HRT) going about their early morning chores - cooking breakfast and getting the family off to work - were in for a shock. Yet another damning report claimed that HRT - which was part of their daily routine - increased the likelihood of dying from breast cancer. It is hard to imagine a worse beginning to a day.

Almost immediately government experts issued an alert to GPs which resulted in HRT prescriptions being refused for women who had been using it for five years or more. NHS help lines were ringing off the hook as women demanded to know whether their health had been put at risk. They besieged GPs surgeries but GPs weren't much help. They, after all, were only responding to the alert dumped on them by the Committee on Safety of Medicines (CSM).

This decision was so badly handled that the Deputy Chief Medical Officer for England was forced to step in to try to quell women's fears that HRT was harmful. But it was too late. GPs had already complied with instructions, put up the shutters and refused to renew HRT prescriptions for women who had been using HRT for more than five years, leaving a million women in the lurch. The whole episode was a complete medical and political cock-up but it served to raise the profile of the charity making the allegations and undoubtedly generated a flood of new donations into their coffers.

Breast cancer charities have caused more harm to women's health by constantly harping on about HRT than any good they might have done to improve treatment for breast cancer. There is no medical-based evidence that HRT harms women. On the contrary, it protects them from a range of diseases of old age.

HRT has become the Aunt Sally for almost every kind of medical research organisation seeking publicity in newspapers and almost everything, from eating grape skins to left-handedness, allegedly doubles the chance of developing breast cancer. More column inches are devoted to it than almost any other form of treatment and most of it is misguided if not downright misleading. **HRT is not a new treatment.** It has been around for almost a century and millions of women the world over, including me, have benefited enormously. But this doesn't seem to discourage publicity seekers from regularly having a pop at it. Even the Medicines and Healthcare Products Regulatory Agency – another government quango – has jumped on the bandwagon. Is it any wonder that women are beginning to question the safety of HRT?

All new ideas meet with resistance, especially when the effects are remarkable and beneficial as they are with HRT. But as a result of this Study, women are told to put up with the menopause just like their mothers and their grandmothers. But very few of our grandmothers lived long enough to suffer the worst of it. In 1900 the average life expectancy of women was 51, today it is nearly 80. The question is whether you are prepared to take an outside chance that none of the problems of old age will affect you or be guaranteed 30 years of relatively good health by replacing missing hormones.

There is still a wide range of views about the benefits and risks of HRT, even within the medical profession. In my opinion, the possible risks have been wildly exaggerated whilst the benefits have been underplayed. And, as a result, many women are suffering unnecessarily - afraid to accept treatment despite its long track record of success. From my personal experience and that of thousands of other women there is nothing as effective in protecting your health and improving your well-being as you grow older. Age becomes irrelevant for women on HRT.

A Publicist's dream

When the public relation's department of a cancer charity sits down to think of some way to raise money from the public they think of breasts. Breasts will guarantee a good size space in the tabloids and, if the allegations are outrageous enough, the story may end up on the front page - every PR department's dream. The fear of breast cancer has become the biggest cash cow for certain cancer charities. It attracts more publicity than almost any other story when, in fact, the risk of breast cancer in older women is extremely low and there is no clear evidence linking it to HRT. Even the Million Women Study said as much – if you bothered to read the small print.

I don't wish to do down all cancer charities for many of which I have the greatest respect, including MacMillan Cancer Relief, who do a wonderful work providing practical and emotional support for cancer patients and their families. But there is no excuse for other cancer charities to play on people's fear.

Meanwhile, the 'Cinderella' cancers affecting colons, testicles, ovaries, wombs and penises, are at the 'boot sale' end of the publicity market. The forgotten 'army' that nobody wants to illustrate on the front page of the tabloids or on the TV.

LINDA'S LETTER

Dear Mrs. Gorman,

I am writing in connection with the news that HRT causes breast cancer and should only be used short term. I am extremely concerned about this as I feel nothing new has been found from this latest Million Women Report; and to call this a 'lifestyle' drug is both ignorant and insulting to all women. I myself thought long and hard before I took the decision to start HRT. I tried all the alternatives plus exercise – but they had no effect.

I didn't have hot flushes or night sweats but my symptoms were horrendous over 4 years. I endured muscle and joint pains to the point where I could hardly walk. The depression and anxiety were impossible to describe and totally debilitating. I started getting migraine for the first time in my life, which caused temporary blindness and weakness in my right side for up to 10 days after each attack. The doctors thought at first that I was suffering mini strokes, as my attacks were so severe. Finally, I lost my voice. My throat became so painful I feared for what it may be. Still I hesitate to go on HRT. After 4 years of these symptoms and 18 months of being mute, I made an intelligent and informed decision to try HRT.

After 12 months of finding the right one for me, all my symptoms melted away. I have my voice back, no vision disturbances or migraine and can exercise again.

I wish to stay on HRT long term and feel incensed that this decision has been taken away from me.

Linda's letter - and others like it - prompted me to write this book to refute allegations made in the Press that HRT is linked to breast cancer in older women. Breast cancer is not caused by using HRT. On the contrary, HRT protects women from many serious diseases of old age and it will be a tragedy if women are forced to give it up.

Chapter 2
THE REAL BREAST CANCER STORY

- DNA testing – Men and breast cancer –
- The biology of breast cancer

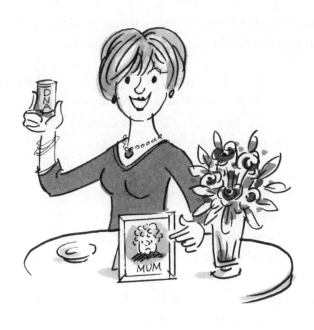

Dear Teresa Gorman

I have been using oestrogen patches plus progestogen for about 11 years. It suits me and I feel good and healthy with the bonus of good skin and hair. My GP normally gives me a supply of HRT for six months at a time, and I also have a mammogram every three years.

On my recent check-up I was told that there are now strict guidelines on HRT and that the risk of breast cancer increases with age and the length of time one is on it.

I realise it is important to protect against illnesses but breast cancer does not run in my family. Despite this, the doctor refused me further treatment. Therefore, knowing you approve of HRT, and look great on it, I turn to you and ask please can you arm me with some positive information to put to my doctor in support of my needs.

It seems we have no say if the GP refuses to prescribe it and this scares me so much. My only hope is to fight with valid arguments. I'd be most grateful for any help and advice you could offer me. Please, please help.

Extract from a letter from Patricia T.

Women who are forced to give up HRT are in real danger. Not only may their menopause symptoms return with a vengeance but also serious diseases, including osteoporosis and heart attacks, begin to accelerate. The risk of erratic behaviour and depression, which can cause the breakdown of a marriage, can also be due to the lack of female hormones.

The latest research indicates that breast cancer runs in families. If you are unlucky enough to have inherited the risk, there is evidence to show that HRT – as used by older women - *delays* the onset of the disease by about 10 years. More than that, it also protects women from other inevitable problems of growing old, including brittle bones, a dickey heart and going gaga. And if you read the small print of The Million Women Report it says much the same thing.

It is always a tragedy when a young woman dies of breast cancer. But, when the tabloid newspapers feature stories about breast cancer, they almost always feature young women and neglect to point out that young women don't take HRT.

From puberty young women are awash with female hormones and their breast tissue is highly sensitive to oestrogen – the female hormone which is held responsible for causing breast cancer. Even so, not every young woman develops breast cancer. This indicates that there is some other agent at work. Hormone replacement as used by older women simply replaces hormones – *but by a much smaller amount* – just enough to keep your body in good working order.

So, you can forget the scare stories linking breast cancer and HRT. If you have reached the menopause without developing breast cancer, it is much less likely you will develop breast cancer and only if you have inherited the tendency. Based on the available evidence, in my view it is wrong to suggest that the tiny amount of hormones in HRT will harm you. Indeed, the evidence now is very strong that HRT started below the age of 60 particularly if it is oestrogen alone (without progestogen) does show a decrease in breast cancer and a decrease in heart attacks.

DNA testing

Breast cancer runs in families but not all women know their family history. DNA testing will soon solve this problem. A DNA test can detect the risk of developing breast cancer by examining a few cells taken with a swab from the inside of the mouth. This service will soon be available at your GP's surgery. In the meantime, there are many companies offering this service on the Internet. It couldn't be simpler. They send you a home testing kit which you return to them for analysis. This test is especially appropriate for young women if breast cancer runs in their family. The sooner the risk is identified, the easier it is to control.

Older women can benefit from having a DNA test if they are worried about developing breast cancer and for them, regular breast screening makes sense. At present, breast screening is only available to women between the ages of 50 and 64 but cancer can develop later. If you have been lucky enough to escape breast cancer while you were young the risk is extremely low until you reach your 70s when *'they are smaller, localised cancers, easy to cure and rarely fatal'*, says Professor Valerie Beral, Director of the Million Women Study.

As people grow older - men and women alike – we are more likely to develop diseases of old age. The good news is that scientists can already identify many of the genes responsible so that we can take action before a disease becomes a problem. DNA testing will revolutionise our understanding of cancer – and other diseases – so that they can be treated before they become life-threatening. Which raises the question of what we will die of – probably boredom - or because the money runs out!

Men and breast cancer

Men, too, develop breast cancer and the sons of male cancer victims are six times more likely to develop the disease. Which reinforces the evidence that breast cancer is hereditary and you don't need female hormones to develop the disease.

The biology of breast cancer

Breast cancer is now one of the most widely studied diseases in the world. For those who would like to know more about this research Dr. Amineh Abbu Zayyad, a leading analyst of genetics, has carried out an extensive survey of the biology of breast cancer studies and an extract from her research is given at Appendix I at the end of this book.

Chapter 3
ALL ABOUT HRT

How hormones work – Testosterone is a girl's best friend - What is HRT? – HRT and your general health – HRT and your mental health – Five years is not enough - What happens if you stop taking HRT – Why do women give up HRT?

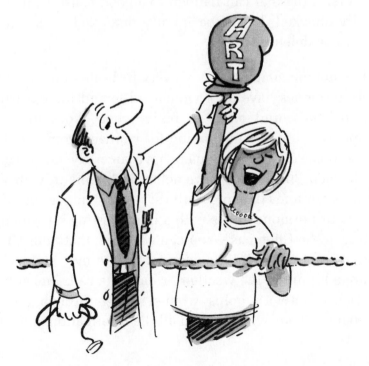

Dear Ms Gorman,

I just wanted to say how pleased I was to read your support of HRT in a recent newspaper. I am 55 years of age and have been using HRT since the start of an early menopause at the age of 41 after giving birth to my son. My symptoms were aching hands and neck making it almost impossible to get my head off the pillow in the morning. After discovering that I had an incredibly low hormone level my doctor put me onto HRT without delay. I haven't looked back until now when my GP tells me I can no longer have HRT. What am I to do now?

Letter from Sarah W.

The worst thing that can happen to a good cause is, not to be skilfully attacked, but to be ineptly defended – and no one seems to be defending HRT.

Sarah is not unusual in knowing very little about the influence which hormones have on a woman's life and the devastating effect on the mind and the body when they run out at menopause. It is not uncommon for younger women to begin the menopause. Some women have an early menopause – even in their 30s. If you have aches and pains in your joints or other symptoms like forgetfulness or bad temper you should check your hormone levels with a home testing kit which you can buy at the Chemists. You can't assume that your GP will automatically recognise the symptoms. He may just feel that you are a bit under the weather or having a bad time at home. The Daisy Network helps women going through an early menopause. They will give you all the information and advice you need. The address to write to is: The Daisy Network, PO Box 183, Rossendale, BB4 6WZ.

How hormones work

Hormones are a kind of telegraph system running between your brain and your body, making sure they work in harmony and it will help to understand why there are good days and bad days.

The two key hormones are oestrogen (pronounced ee-stro-gen) - which makes you feel energetic and enthusiastic about life while progestogen (pronounced pro-jesto-jen) has the opposite effect. They determine your femininity and your ability to conceive. But your flirtatious behaviour towards the opposite sex is controlled by the small - but significant - amount of testosterone, usually thought of as the male hormone. All three hormones are directly related to your role in producing the next generation which is what nature designed you for.

As menopause approaches, your natural supply of these hormones begins to run down and confused messages are sent between your body and your brain causing absent-mindedness, moods and depression. People close to you will notice changes in your behaviour even though you may not be aware of the cause.

Menopause marks the end of your fertility but it need not interfere with the rest of your life so long as you take control of it. By replacing the missing hormones you can even turn this time of your life into an opportunity for a fresh start. Women often say that HRT gives them a new lease of life – to do what they always wanted to do - but lacked the self-confidence to do it.

Testosterone is a girl's best friend

Testosterone is the latest addition to hormone replacement and is fantastic stuff *for women*. It's not just men who need testosterone – it puts the 'X' factor back into your sex life when it is not uncommon for women in their 30s and 40s to lose interest in the sexual side of their relationship and testosterone makes you more lively, self-confident and competitive at work. And, so long as you are taking it with your HRT it won't make you grow whiskers on your chin.

Ever since I became an MP I've had a testosterone implant every six months when I have my HRT renewed. It was originally recommended to me by my gynaecologist who rightly said that I would need it to stand up to the bully-boys in the debating chamber and battle it out with testosterone-driven male MPs. It definitely boosted my energy levels, memory and the ability to think on my feet. And, even though I have given up politics, I still take it and nothing on earth would persuade me to give it up.

The latest testosterone products in the pipeline include a gel, a cream and a spray, as well as a pill. And it is also available in a 'patch' to use alongside your HRT patch. It restores the confidence which women begin to lose with menopause - at just the point in their lives when they have more time to devote to themselves and maybe start a whole new career. You will have a much better chance of making a success of whatever you choose to do if you are in control of your body's hormones instead of letting them dictate to you.

Testosterone makes all the difference to women who are working in a man's world especially when you find yourself in confrontational situations. Women are usually the first to back down in these situations but testosterone will enable you to stand up for yourself.

What is HRT?

When women say they feel so much better on HRT, that's because of the oestrogen effect. So why take progestogen? Because it safeguards the lining of the womb. More about that later.

HRT is a remarkably simple form of treatment and incredibly cheap. It also protects you from the more serious diseases of old age, the risk from which accelerates after menopause. The practice of replacing hormones is widely used in medicine for all sorts of other hormone-related problems such as diabetes, thyroid deficiency and abnormal growth in children, to mention just a few. It is a well-known fact that the ointment, which is rubbed into the fetlocks of horses, contains a high level of oestrogen to protect their skeletons. The unexpected side effect is that women who work with horses have remarkably fine complexions, having absorbed the oestrogen through their skin! No one bats an eyelid about the many uses of hormones – except when it comes to HRT for women. This tells you more about the prejudice that surrounds middle age in women than it does about concern for their health.

HRT and your general health

Your female hormones not only control the reproductive part of your life, they also boost your immune system delaying serious medical problems associated with old age. It is a well-known fact in medical circles that a high level of oestrogen in young women accounts for the fact that their general health is better than that of young men. In her book No Change, Wendy Cooper describes an American health study involving 50,000 older women which found that replacing hormones not only improved general health but it also delayed the onset of serious diseases of old age, such as heart attacks and even breast cancer, by an average of 10 years.

HRT and your mental health

Oestrogen also keeps you mentally alert for longer so that you continue to enjoy an active life and enables you to remain independent. It stimulates the growth and replacement of brain cells without which you become absentminded as you grow older and, eventually, develop Alzheimer's disease. Current medical advice to stop taking HRT after 5 or 10 years is thoroughly misguided when you think of all the awful things that can happen to you if you do.

Oestrogen enables your body to renew itself - which is why women who use HRT have good complexions, are physically fit, and enjoy a better quality of life. If your doctor recommends you give it up tell him or her politely that you have no intention of doing so because it would be like giving up on life itself!

Five years is not enough

Taking HRT for just five years as recommended by the Committee on Safety of Medicine is not nearly long enough. Your symptoms will return and you will start to go through the menopause all over again but, more seriously, you deprive yourself of the long-term benefits. Only this time you are five years older and the physical effects (damage) may be worse. If the government won't pay for it, women should at least be able to buy it for themselves – it's not all that expensive. But why do women allow themselves to be treated like this? It is another sign of the contempt in which women are held in our society – older women in particular – but it doesn't have to be so. Pick up your pen and write to your Member of Parliament. Every woman has a vote – and that's what counts to MPs.

What happens if you stop taking HRT?

With increasing age your menopause symptoms may subside but I have known women who suffered from hot flushes right through into their 70s. HRT can certainly give you a break from that possibility. But there is no health reason why you should ever give it up. On the contrary, there are many women in their 70s who still use HRT – I'm one of them - and we are remarkably alert and active for our age.

The constant use of HRT that protects against heart disease and osteoporosis, so it's no good giving it up after five years as the government recommends. Women who begin to use HRT at the onset of menopause reduce the risk of coronary heart disease by 30% but the benefit diminishes the longer women you are without it. In other words, the earlier you begin to take HRT the better your heart is protected, according to the American Journal of Women's Health.

Why do women give up HRT?

When hormone replacement has so many advantages why are so few women using it? There are ten and a half million women in this country that could benefit yet half the women who begin to use HRT give up within six to nine months. The side effects, such as a mini 'period', feeling bloated or breast tenderness, puts some women off. Even more women are unnecessarily discouraged by fear of developing breast cancer when HRT has nothing at all to do with it.

I think you should stop worrying about possible side effects which are really minor – or non-existent – and start thinking of what benefits you can gain by keeping up the level of your female hormones.

Chapter 4
TYPES OF HRT TREATMENT

*HRT treatments - The HRT pill - The skin patch –
Oestrogel - Oestrogen creams - Implants - Progestogen
– the side effects - The Mirena ring - HRT and the
contraceptive pill*

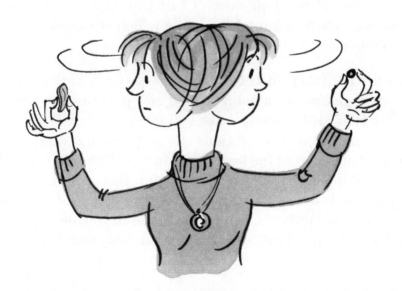

> *"HRT should not be withheld from post-menopausal women, since there is no evidence that the small amount of oestrogen in HRT increases their risk of breast cancer while added progestogen significantly reduces risk of cancer of the womb"*, says Professor John Studd, a leading Consultant on HRT who gave me the benefit of his long experience in this field when writing this book.

When it comes to HRT we are spoiled for choice but how many of us know it? HRT comes in numerous forms: pills, patches, implants, gels or even a nasal spray and if you want to know more about them you can look it up on the Internet.

The basic hormone you need is oestrogen but the other female hormone, progestogen, is recommended as a precaution to prevent the build up of the lining of the womb. Different manufacturers provide various combinations of these two hormones and it is largely a matter of trial and error as to what suits you. If one type doesn't suit you, you can always try another. There is bound to be one which is right for you, so don't give up.

It's the oestrogen in HRT which gives you a 'lift' while the progestogen causes a 'mini' period and puts some women off using HRT. HRT should make you feel better but, if it doesn't come up your expectations it is probably due to the progestogen part of the treatment. In which case, ask your GP for a different type. It's important that you know and understand the pros and cons of the types of treatment available and then you can have a say in the matter, especially if the first type of HRT you are given doesn't suit you.

The HRT pill

Of all the ways of taking HRT, the simplest, cheapest and most convenient is in the form of a pill which is taken every day. There are several types –

a) Oestrogen-only pill suitable for women who have had their womb removed.

b) Combined HRT packs which consists of two types of pills – oestrogen and progestogen – taken in sequence.

c) Continuous HRT in which each pill contains a mixture of oestrogen and progestogen

Different brands come in different combinations – some from natural sources, some made in the laboratory – which gives a wide choice with the ability to swap around until you find one which is right for you.

The skin patch

Some women find it difficult to remember to take a pill each day but the patch only has to be replaced twice a week. It costs more than the pill and, for this reason, your GP may be reluctant to prescribe it. The patch is about the size of a 50p piece and you stick it on your bottom where it remains for several days at a time. If it comes off in the shower or in bed you can stick it on again. If you put it in the same place each time it may irritate your skin so you will have to move it around.

The patch contains oestrogen dissolved in a solvent, which passes through your skin directly into the blood stream reducing the risk of liver problems and gallstones. Because the patch costs more women are sometimes recommended to switch to the pill. So be sure to question your GP if he suggests you should do so and, if necessary, ask him to make a check to see that this decision will not carry any risk for you.

The latest development is a patch containing the male hormone testosterone a little of which your body makes when you are young. Already dubbed 'pink Viagra' and a marriage saver, it beefs up your self-confidence and your love life. You will still need a prescription from your GP to obtain it and you will probably have to pay for it yourself.

Oestrogel

When I first went to my doctor with menopause symptoms he recommended HRT in the form of a gel to spread round my middle after a morning shower. Apparently, this form of HRT is favoured by French women who think nothing of strolling around the bedroom stark naked while it dries. Alternatively, try using a hairdryer to speed things up. Today it comes in neat foil packets – one a day – or in a pump. I still keep a supply by me just in case my implant runs down before the six months is up. Oestrogel is also used as an antidote for migraine which can be caused by too much progestogen in your system. It is even recommended for young women who suffer towards the end of their monthly period from pre-menstrual tension – or post-menstrual depression. Either way it can cure your 'period' blues.

Oestrogen creams

Even if you have an easy menopause and you have ruled out taking HRT, you may still want to continue in a sexual relationship even though the skin lining your vagina becomes thin and dry. Oestrogen cream, another product available on the Internet, can cure the problem but make sure you buy one which includes *oestrodiol* and is not made from yams which, according to Professor Studd, a leading gynaecologist and HRT specialist, does not have the desired effect.

Implants

Once you have settled down with HRT you may wish to consider an implant - which is much more convenient - but you will have to pay for a gynaecologist to insert it for you. An implant lasts from six months to a year so you don't have to think about it every day. If you want to give it a try this method you can ask your GP to refer you to a gynaecologist but you will probably have to pay as a private patient. Alternatively, telephone a PPP or BUPA hospital and ask for an appointment with a gynaecologist. Be sure to ask about the fee for both the consultation and the implant before you book.

The implant consists of a tiny oestrogen pellet, about the size of an apple pip, popped under the skin just above the bikini line. You don't have to remove all your clothes to have it done and the whole procedure only takes a few minutes. It is pretty painless but some Consultants uses a local anaesthetic. You can also ask for a testosterone implant at the same time to soup up your lovelife. I have been having an implant for 20 years and you can take my word for it, you will be firing on all cylinders.

Don't forget to make a note in your diary to remind yourself when your next implant is due. Implants should last for 6 months but they sometimes begin to fade before then and you may be aware that you are not feeling quite so wide awake as usual. I begin to yawn a lot so I pick up the telephone to make my next appointment – and, meanwhile, I use oestrogel to keep me going. It saves having an argument with your gynaecologist who may be reluctant to renew your implant early.

Progestogen – the side effects

The progestogen part of HRT, which is recommended to prevent the build-up of the lining of the womb - can produce mood swings - 5% to 10% of women HRT users are highly susceptible. Some women also object to having a period caused by progestogen which can be heavy if the amount of progestogen is too high. You can adjust the amount yourself - without bothering your GP. And you may only need to take progestogen every three months or so - just to be on the safe side.

Another downside to progestogen is water retention and other undesirable effects similar to bloating and breast tenderness which women experience just before a period. In which case, reduce the dose. It can also cause the occasional migraine headache or cramp in the legs, both of which commonly occur in young women before a period when their progestogen level is high. As a temporary measure try taking a couple of tablets for a headache and 'Crampex' tablets if you get cramp in your legs. Tailoring progestogen to suit your needs is the best way to deal with these problems. Progestogen intolerance is very important. It is a major reason why some women stop taking HRT. The trick is to reduce the dose, reduce the duration or to change the progestogen. Here are some other suggestions passed on to me by gynaecologists which you might like to try:

Avoid tablets containing the combined form of HRT - change to a prescription which provides oestrogen and progestogen separately which enables you to adjust the dose. For example:

❖ Take progestogen for 5 days instead of the recommended 10 and see if this is sufficient to produce a mini period, (which may not occur for several days after you have stopped taking progestogen).

❖   Take progestogen every other day.

❖   For long-term users of HRT, try taking it once every three
    months which is what I do. Ideally, progestogen should
    be tailored to suit your needs. I take my progestogen
    overnight to which means you sleep through any adverse
    effects and I have rarely have any trouble.

The Mirena ring

The Mirena 'ring' gives out a tiny amount of progestogen each
day which keeps the lining of the womb clear and is
recommended as a treatment for women who don't get on with
progestogen taken by mouth or for women who don't want to
continue with 'periods' after the menopause. The ring, which
is available on the advice of a gynaecologist, is inserted into
the vagina, similar to the contraceptive coil. Professor John
Studd, a leading gynaecologist, has this to say about it,

> *"It has proved highly successful with the majority of my
> patients and I strongly recommend it. It has transformed
> menopause therapy and, at the same time, reduced the
> need for a   hysterectomy by 50%. But, it can be easily
> removed if you don't get on with it"*.

You should expect to have some teething troubles when you
first take HRT and you should be able to iron them out by
talking to your GP or your consultant. HRT is not a 'one size
fits all' product. It's more like buying a pair of shoes; you may
need to try several different kinds before you find one you are
comfortable with. So persevere – because you're worth it!

HRT is refused to older women who have been diagnosed with
breast cancer and had a breast removed. Instead they are given
radiography followed by chemotherapy to destroy any cancer

still in their system. And as a result, tiredness, depression and terrible night sweats return. But, if you accept the view that HRT has nothing to do with the development of breast cancer in older women, there is really no reason why you should be put through this misery.

HRT and the contraceptive pill

Some women confuse HRT with the undesirable side effects once attributed to the contraceptive pill. *The two are completely different.* HRT replaces the natural supply of hormones that you lose when menopause begins. The contraceptive pill was designed to repress the production of a monthly egg cell and so prevent you from becoming pregnant. There are millions of women worldwide who have used the Pill for many years without problems and today it is even prescribed for teenagers to prevent unwanted pregnancies. That still doesn't prevent it from coming in for some bogus criticism even though – or perhaps because – it enables women to control their fertility which, deep down, is resented by some of the men who rule the world.

HRT is another of the great advances in medicine, on a par with penicillin and the contraceptive pill. All three have saved many women's lives and protected women from many fatal diseases. No one in their right mind would dream of suggesting that penicillin is an affront to nature and I cannot recall anything in the whole of history that has been more beneficial to women than HRT other than antibiotics and the contraceptive pill, both of which transformed women's lives.

Chapter 5
YOU AND YOUR GP

*When Doctor says 'No' - The doctor's dilemma
and the compensation culture – Walk-in centres –
Alternative therapies and the 'natural' route –
Feminists and Agony Aunts*

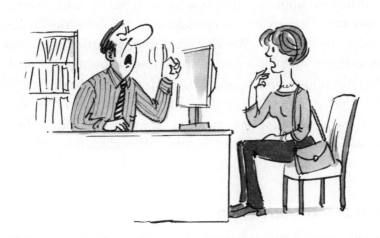

Dear Teresa Gorman,

I have read that one woman in five suffers no ill effects from the menopause. That 'one' is very fortunate, but it leaves the rest of us to have a grim old time unless we are very fortunate in our choice of GP. My own doctor cannot truly have been described as hostile. He responded to my catalogue of miseries – just the usual ones but no more bearable for that – with a smirking indifference. It was not easy in a small community to change doctors. I am a person who hates confrontation, but I felt I had no choice. It was the best move I could have made. My new GP is a middle-aged woman who not only understands my symptoms, she has them too and we both use ART!

Letter from Joanna D.

The thinnest book in the world is what men know about women and, if men had a menopause, HRT would be dished out with the rations. We live in a man's world but, even so, women themselves are partly to blame for being so timid and apologetic about menopause. Anything that is done to stop women obtaining HRT will, ultimately, add to the cost of health care because as women grow older they become seriously incapacitated and in need of constant medical care. Penny wise, pound foolish.

When Doctor says 'No'

"I have been going through hell, but I think my doctor's attitude was 'do the benefits for you, right now, outweigh the risks?' How am I to answer that?", asks another of my correspondents.

Before the MWS, most GPs would have prescribed HRT knowing full well that their patients benefitted. Some doctors still feel that the possible risks of HRT have been wildly exaggerated and that many women suffer unnecessarily because they are now afraid to accept treatment that is guaranteed to work. However sympathetic your GP may or may not be, he may not have a detailed knowledge of HRT or know how to adapt it to your personal needs.

Ultimately they take their orders from the government who control the products they are allowed to prescribe and sets their budget and targets - just as they once did in communist countries. We are the only country left in the Western world which has this antiquated system. When women write to me to say that their GP refuses to renew their prescription after five years they can, in fact, buy it over the Internet or see a gynaecologist privately. It is easier than changing your GP.

My advice is to try to avoid having open warfare with your doctor - you catch more flies with honey than with vinegar. Emphasise that you are not prepared to put up with the return of your menopause symptoms, which interfere with your work, the quality of your life and that of your family.

If all else fails, it is possible under the NHS rules to change your doctor and, however reluctant you may be to do so, you have a vested interest in your health. However, this is easier said than done. In rural areas it can be almost impossible. In which case, you can ask for a second opinion to which you are entitled under NHS rules. Feeling well is not an option but a necessity; so don't be afraid of combining your tact with firmness.

The doctor's dilemma and the compensation culture

The Million Women Study (MWS) led to GPs limiting HRT prescriptions to the first five years but all this does is delay the onset of menopause symptoms and this gives GPs a powerful reason for turning down your request for long-term treatment. Financial considerations also influence the type of HRT you are likely to be offered – usually pills – which don't suit everyone. GPs, who are inclined to take a 'wait-and-see' attitude to menopause, are much more likely to be unsympathetic towards women who wish to continue with HRT after the first five years. This simply delays the onset of serious health problems including osteoporosis (brittle bone disease), heart attacks and strokes and these diseases kill far more women at an earlier age than breast cancer.

Some GPs simply don't take the long-term effects of untreated menopause seriously. The suggestion that five years of HRT are sufficient to see you through menopause is quite wrong. And the Press, from which most women get their information, simply reports surveys which blow hot and cold. All this plays fast and loose with your health. It's no wonder that women don't know what to believe or which way to turn.

Governments consistently put too low a priority on the health of older women while GPs fear that if they go against government advice they risk becoming the victims of the compensation culture.

Walk-in centres

An alternative for women who are having difficulties with their GP would be the development of walk-in multi-screening centres where women could get a check-up without being referred by their GP. They could be based in breast screening centres which could be adapted to offer regular health checks for women over 50 on a variety of age-related health problems. This would include:

1. DNA test for the risk of developing breast cancer. The DNA test requires a few cells taken with a mouth swab which is like a cotton bud. This is sent to a laboratory to be checked and the results can be produced within a matter of hours.

2. Blood pressure and cholesterol test to establish the risk for heart disease. A blood pressure test only requires you to roll up your sleeve and a cholesterol test requires a blood sample.

3. Ultra-sound or DEXA scan to check for osteoporosis. Bone scanning by ultra-sound is a simple matter. You only have to remove your shoe and stocking and a result comes up on a computer screen.

DEXA scans are more sophisticated and expensive and are not yet freely available on the NHS. It is preferable to have a bone scan *before* menopause so that you have a record of the structure of your bones which can then be compared with later scans, particularly if you are *not* taking HRT.

All these tests are simple, quick and painless - and a lot more pleasant than having your breasts regularly squashed in the scanning machine!

Alternative therapies and the 'natural' route

"I have spent the last two years studying the fashionable plant hormone, phyto-oestrogen, but it is not absorbed and it does not have any effect except possibly helps anxiety, but even that is doubtful". John Studd, Professor of Gynaecology, Chelsea & Westminster Hospital.

Some women believe menopause is a natural event and we should accept it. So is short sight, receding gums and increasing deafness, but no one would dream of suggesting that you should put up with these. For women who object to using 'drugs' (HRT is *not* a drug), there are plant products which are not controlled and, where their effects have been scientifically studied, are not effective. They can also be very expensive. If the experience of women recently deprived of HRT prescriptions is anything to go by, these alternatives don't work. Take a look at the 'chatter' on the Internet between women swapping horror stories about the return of menopause symptoms and asking for advice. The overwhelming balance of opinion is that they don't work.

Others swear by vitamins E & C, which are found in all kinds of nuts and seeds. Ginseng, which contains plant 'oestrogen', has been used for centuries to relieve 'women's troubles'. There are other herbs that some women put their faith in. But nothing relieves menopause symptoms as effectively as the oestrogen in HRT which millions of women, world wide, can testify to. The effect is almost miraculous. Hot flushes disappear and they feel wonderful again. Tranquillisers and other pick-me-up treatments may have a short-term effect but your symptoms will return. Many women who experience sleeping problems at menopause may be prescribed sleeping pills which work for a short time but the body eventually builds up a tolerance to them – and then you are back to square one again. A glass of warm milk can be just as effective.

Feminists and Agony Aunts

The popular TV presenter Gloria Hunniford champions 'natural' methods to combat menopause symptoms. There is a whole literature of advice on diet and plant materials to combat hot flushes, memory loss and other symptoms for women who prefer to try the natural route. I have no practical experience and cannot comment.

Germaine Greer - our national and almost only post-menopausal female intellectual to appear regularly on TV and radio - is so strongly opposed to HRT that she sat down and wrote a *whole* book, in which she attacked me for recommending it to other women. Germaine thinks that growing old naturally – wrinkles and all - has some particular virtue. In her book she depicts me as a traitor to the feminist cause. She objected to my promotion of HRT because it undermined the dignity of older women who should be allowed to grow old gracefully. No mention of ill health. HRT has a beneficial effect on your temper as well as your judgement and I regularly recommend it to women for this very reason. What is noble about growing old 'naturally' as Germaine recommends when it means ending up, crippled, incontinent, bad-tempered and even gaga?

You should make up your own mind which path to follow – Germaine's, Gloria's or mine? What matters is that the choice is yours – not a feminist, an agony aunt, or even your local GP.

Chapter 6
MENOPAUSE SYMPTOMS AND RELATED DISEASES

Palpitations and hot flushes – Painful Joints - Vaginitis, cystitis and thrush – Incontinence - Checklist of menopause symptoms – Heart attacks and strokes – Osteoporosis – the silent disease – The scanning process

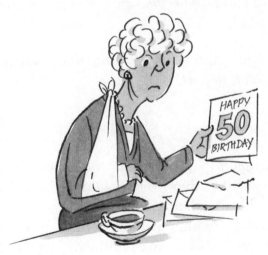

Dear Teresa Gorman,

"At 44 my periods fizzled out. I was engulfed in hot flushes very rapidly. My GP was sympathetic but reluctant to act upon her knowledge. She sent me to the local hospital. The female consultant was impatient with me. She described my symptoms to my GP as mere 'panic attacks'. I also had vaginal dryness and no period bleeding.

At that time I was an infant school teacher. The school Head knew I was a good teacher, but suddenly I was becoming a dud one. I became distressed and alarmed. I had constant headaches. My husband scored high marks for sympathy. Yet it was not cups of tea I needed, it was HRT.

If I had not insisted on plain answers I would have been fobbed off with sleeping pills. HRT has been such a godsend for me that I am exasperated by the allegations against it. I can't argue the science. I just know I'm living proof it works".

Letter received from Mary H. after the publication of the Million Women Report.

In the past, women like Mary kept their menopause a secret because it meant that they were no longer young and fertile and even risked losing their job or their partner – discarded for a younger model - which still happens. But today, when women have the means to avoid the worst aspects of menopause blues by using HRT they are not allowed to make this decision for themselves. It's the government that decides.

Palpitations and hot flushes

If a middle-aged man has 'palpitations' he is likely to be rushed into hospital in case he is having a heart attack. But a middle-aged woman is more likely to be offered a cup of tea because her symptoms would be considered to be due to menopause. This perfectly illustrates the difference in attitude towards danger signs in women and men. It is not generally recognised that a heart attack is the principal cause of death in older woman – forty times more common than breast cancer.

Painful joints

Painful joints caused by arthritis and rheumatism is also associated with your skeleton and is a long-term health problem affecting 7 million people, three-quarters of them women. The symptoms tend to begin in the small joints, such as fingers and toes, followed by pain and swelling in other joints. The pain tends to improve during pregnancy which suggests that female hormones may be involved.

You may be one of those lucky women who escape hot flushes, palpitations and other symptoms which creep up and zap you. In my case it was a sudden loss of memory and aches and pains in my joints. They were so painful that, when cooking, I couldn't use a knife to slice things or walk up the stairs carrying the laundry because my ankles hurt so much.

I was still in my early 40s when I started to nod off at my desk in the office. And, although I was unaware of it, I yawned so much that my secretary began to suspect I was having a secret affair that kept me up nights! Finally, I took myself off to Chelsea Women's Hospital thinking I was losing my mind. Thank goodness they recognised the symptoms.

They recommended HRT and I have been as right as nine pence ever since.

Vaginitis, cystitis and thrush

This is *not* the name of the latest 'pop' group and it's a lot less fun! These are three of the most common complaints which are almost guaranteed to turn up in post-menopausal women and can be very painful and embarrassing because they make you itch.

Vaginitis occurs as a result of the lining of the vagina drying out, losing its natural antiseptic qualities. Taking HRT keeps skin healthy both inside and outside your body and prevents this problem.

Cystitis - sometimes called the 'honeymoon disease' can be caught during sexual intimacy or from germs from the back passage. Either way, it can infect the bladder and even the kidneys. Jenny Murray who presents Woman's Hour on the BBC told me that their programme on cystitis brought in the biggest postbag they had ever received – apart from the one on HRT – which indicates that it is a very common complaint. You can now treat it yourself with tablets available 'over the counter'.

Thrush is a nice name for a nasty fungus that also thrives in your plumbing region and makes you itch like mad. It is common to all ages and can be caught from sexual contact or a reaction to soap or shower gel. You can use an antibiotic cream, which is available from the chemist to deal with the itching problem and choose cotton underwear, not those non-absorbent, synthetic, thongy things which are likely to make things worse.

Incontinence

Incontinence is not funny. If you look on the shelves of your local Chemist at the packets of incontinence pads you realise that stress incontinence – leaking – is extremely common problem for women. In middle-aged women the cause is a weakening of the bladder muscles which is less likely to happen if you take HRT.

Leaking can happen if you cough, sneeze or laugh too enthusiastically. Squeezing the muscles between your legs can help to strengthen the bladder which is an exercise you can perform while watching TV or standing at the bus stop.

We are born doubly incontinent, without hair or teeth and by the time you reach old age you may be back where you started. You may end up wearing more padding than a pair of baby Pampers. From nappies to nappies. I don't know how much the NHS spends on padded underwear for women but I guess it is costing a small fortune. The only way to escape these indignities is by using HRT to keep up your oestrogen levels. In Japan some remarkable research into the health problems of old age proved that even senile women could regain muscle control if they are given HRT.

Checklist of menopause symptoms

Here is a checklist of the more common menopause symptoms: This list is not exhaustive. Take a look on the Internet where women left stranded by the MWS air their views. If your symptoms have returned don't suffer in silence. Some doctors have relented and reinstated HRT prescriptions.

Physical Symptoms	Mental Performance
Irregular periods	
Hot flushes	lack of concentration
Night sweats	Poor memory
Palpitations of the heart	Lack of self-confidence
Bloating	Insomnia
Bone/joint pain	Mood swings
Dry eyes	
Dry skin	Emotional symptoms
Vaginal dryness	Anxiety
Painful intercourse	Short temper
Hair loss	Panic attacks
Migraine headache	Unable to cope
Sleep problems	Tense and irritable
Breast tenderness	Aggressive
Stress incontinence (leaking)	Suicidal
Itching all over	Depression
Weepy	Lack of interest in sex

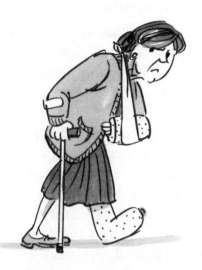

DISEASES CAUSED BY THE MENOPAUSE

"All life is a gamble and if you like to have a flutter then the odds of dying of a heart attack are 2 to 1, osteoporosis is 10 to 1 and breast cancer is a very long shot at 40 to 1. If you regularly use HRT you would be wasting your money on the bet because the chances are the bookie will die before you do".

A fellow Speaker at the International Congress on the Menopause held in Sweden 1993 made this aside to me. It was ironic to be holding the Congress in Sweden because all Swedish women are recommended to use HRT as soon as they come off the contraceptive pill. Menopause is not just a passing phase; it is the beginning of life-threatening diseases and should be taken seriously. There is only one way to reduce the risk and that is to replace the hormones that protected you when you were younger. Female hormones are not just about fertility – they also safeguard your general health.

Heart attacks and strokes

I once attended a debate In Parliament on the subject of growing up without a father, which highlighted the effect that a heart attack can have on a young family which loses a father at an early age. The purpose of the debate was to draw attention to the need for more funding for research into heart disease in young men. When I pointed out that heart attacks kill more middle-aged women than any other disease - and that they, too, may also have a family to look after - my remarks were contemptuously dismissed as a 'feminist intervention'! A heart attack is thought of as a 'man's disease' because it happens to men at a much earlier age, but heart attacks and strokes kill more women over 50 than all the cancers and other diseases of old age put together. HRT also prevents the build up of cholesterol which slows down the flow of blood to the muscles of the heart which is the principal cause of heart attacks. In her book No Change, Wendy Cooper quotes an American health study of 50,000 women which found that taking HRT for 10 years or more halved the number of heart attacks.

Osteoporosis – the silent disease.

"My life has been frantic, what with both hips being replaced eleven months ago and now my wrists needing surgery. The recovery has been remarkable but sometimes I wish I were back on my regular diet of anti-inflammatory drugs that used to mask the ageing of all my other joints. The doctors have me off them now that they have treated my gammy hips." Letter from Margaret in Australia.

This letter came from a personal friend who I failed to persuade to take HRT when she had an early menopause. Now

52, and hobbling about on crutches, she is wondering whether she will be able to fly from Australia to be here for the birth of her first grandchild. If only I had been able to persuade her to take HRT she wouldn't be in this difficulty. Since the advent of HRT osteoporosis has become an optional disease and the tragedy is that so many women have been put off taking it – or denied it by their GPs after five years of treatment at just the time when osteoporosis becomes a serious threat. Women should not allow themselves to be fobbed off with other quack remedies which are totally ineffective.

The National Osteoporosis Society has traditionally been ambivalent in its attitude to HRT, often emphasising alternative remedies such as additional vitamins and calcium-based treatments. However, on their 'Question and Answer' Page on the Society's website, the present Chairman, Professor David Barlow, appears to disagree.

> *"HRT should be seriously considered as an option to effectively alleviate these (menopausal) problems and those women who use HRT for this purpose should have confidence that they are having protection against bone loss and osteoporosis risk at the same time. However when a woman eventually stops HRT, there will again be a loss of bone mass. It is only if HRT is continued for a very long span of years that the skeleton will be sufficiently protected and osteoporotic fractures are likely to be prevented".*

Osteoporosis is called the 'silent disease' because you don't feel anything until your bones begin to break. One in three women over the age of 60 are already suffering from brittle bones but most of them are unaware of it until they accidentally fall and suddenly find themselves with a broken wrist, ankle, or even a hip fracture. This disease is much more common than all of the female cancers put together and second only to heart disease as a cause of early death in middle-aged women.

Early signs of the disease include lower back pain, loss of height, followed by curvature of the spine leading to the development of a Dowager's hump. The President of the NOS, the Duchess of Cornwall, has been at pains to point out that both her mother and grandmother suffered from osteoporosis which indicates that it is an inherited disease - and has little or nothing to do with diet. In severe cases even coughing can cause bones to break - which is why it is called 'brittle bone disease'. But, once you get to this stage, it is usually too late to do much about it. Let us hope that the Duchess takes the advice of the Chairman and takes HRT.

Women who do not use HRT are far more likely to break a bone and because women are more prone to dizzy spells as they grow older they are more likely to fall over and fracture a hip or a wrist. This means an extended stay in hospital because their bones are fragile and may not mend at all. Wear and tear on your joints may result in the need for a hip replacement. A quarter of all women who have this operation die within six months of treatment. Many more can no longer climb the stairs without the aid of a stair lift. But you could carry on ice-skating with HRT if that is your idea of exercise. Mentally, you won't feel old and physically your joints and bones will be strong enough to take the strain.

One of the most depressing features in the weekend press is the pages and pages of adverts for devices to overcome the effects of osteoporosis. Chairs which tilt you forward when you can no longer get on your feet, devices to lower you into the bath and lifts you gently up again, electrically adjustable beds and, when you can no longer walk to the shops, electric scooters. The way to make sure this doesn't happen to you is to protect your bones by taking HRT.

Despite all these advertisements very few women over 50 understand the restricting effect this disease can have on a woman's life when moving around your own home becomes a problem. You may not think it is going to happen to you – but better safe than sorry.

Osteoporosis is another disease which runs in families and second only to heart attack as a frequent cause of death in women over 50. So, if older members of your family have suffered you would be wise to have a DNA test and consider regular bone scans as well as taking HRT.

The scanning process

Middle-aged women are regularly offered breast screening but scanning for osteoporosis is still relatively rare despite the fact that far more women die from the effects of broken bones than from breast cancer. You should ask your GP to refer you for a bone scan as soon as you reach menopause, then you will have a yardstick against which to measure future bone loss.

A DEXA scan is considered to be the 'gold standard' but if it is not yet available in your area then an ultrasound scan probably will be and it can pinpoint those women who are particularly at risk. An ultrasound scan is very simple. It only takes a few seconds and is totally painless. By the time you have put your stocking and shoe back on, the results will be displayed on a small screen so that you can monitor against future scans any bone loss that may have occurred.

Chapter 7
SHOPPING FOR HRT

Girl talk – Going private – BUPA and PPP –
HRT on the Internet – HRT from the Pharmacist

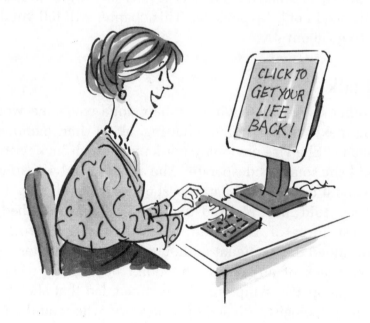

Dear Teresa Gorman,

"If I am refused any more HRT treatment, is it possible to see another GP privately who may agree to prescribe further HRT? I don't know how to find a private doctor and would hope it wasn't too expensive. And I hope it will be treated in confidence. My health and well-being would have to come first. That is my predicament. If you would be kind enough to advise and help me I may well be successful – my husband agrees with me that I should continue with HRT". Extract from a letter from Pamela M.

Pamela's not alone we have all been brought up to rely on the NHS. But, if your GP turns you down, there are plenty of other ways to access HRT and the good news is it need not be expensive. This chapter will tell you how to go about it.

Girl talk

The other day I was having my hair done when the woman sitting next to me began chatting about her menopause problems. She was obviously not having much luck with her GP and she sounded desperate. She asked my advice on what to do about terrible panic attacks she was experiencing. From what she told me I realised that her GP had prescribed the cheapest form of HRT and when that didn't work, he discontinued the treatment without offering her an alternative. GPs are 'jack of all trades' and don't necessarily recognise every menopause symptom. I recommended that she should see a gynaecologist, privately if necessary, who would be able to advise her. And, at that point, I realised just what a problem this could be for a woman with no experience of how to go about it.

When women beg me for advice on something so important to their future health and happiness it really shows that the present system isn't working. Menopause is a major turning point in a woman's life and, in my opinion, access to a specialist is essential. Every woman's experience of menopause is different and treatment should be tailored to the needs of the individual. There are fewer unexpected outcomes if a woman has access to a consultant gynaecologist, who is a specialist in all aspects of female health.

Going private – BUPA and PPP

If your GP still refuses to give you a prescription one alternative is to ask to be referred to a gynaecologist. Almost all gynaecologists will be working in the NHS and you can ask your GP to refer you. But most gynaecologists will be willing to see you privately if you have difficulties with your GP. If you don't want to involve your GP you can phone a private hospital - whether they are BUPA or PPP hospitals - listed in your telephone directory under Private Medical Insurance. When you telephone, ask if they offer a service for menopausal women and make an appointment to see a gynaecologist. *Don't forget to ask about the full cost which will include his or her fee, a charge made by the hospital where the consultation takes place plus a charge for the prescription.* If the consultation takes place in an NHS hospital it will be cheaper than in a private hospital and some gynaecologists are now offering an inclusive service in their own consulting rooms avoiding the charge made by a hospital, making it cheaper and more convenient. The charge will vary in different parts of the country and the type of treatment recommended – pills, patches or an implant - but the annual cost will probably be much less than the amount you spend on cosmetics, clothes or at the hairdressers – and you will get much more of a 'lift' for your money.

Gynaecologists are specialists who are familiar with the full range of menopause symptoms and an up-to-date knowledge of what is on the market - pills, patches, gels, even nasal sprays, and their potential side effects which can vary with the type of prescription you are given. Feel free to discuss your treatment with the gynaecologist as well as the relevant costs of different products. An implant is rarely recommended for a first time user of HRT – although it is much the most convenient method and can last up to a year before it needs to be renewed.

HRT on the Internet

Women are generally good at shopping but when it comes to HRT you are obliged to rely on your GP to make a choice for you and the GP is likely to recommend the cheapest product on the market. Manufacturers of prescription-only drugs are not allowed to advertise their products in the popular press so how can women make an informed choice? This section will enable you to 'shop' for HRT in an informed way and the good news is that you can now buy it via the Internet so, once you have settled down with your prescription – and you may have to try different kinds - you will no longer be at the mercy of your GP and the 'Men from the Ministry'. In the USA you can even consult a specialist via the Internet to discuss the different possibilities and, hopefully, this service will eventually be available to women in the UK.

If you know what your prescription is you can purchase your HRT on the Internet. I recommend you search for UK sites such as **inhousedrugstore.co.uk.** There is no requirement for an online consultation or a doctor's prescription in order to buy online and all prices are in pounds sterling. The order may cost you a little more than a NHS prescription but it is much more convenient. And, you have a choice on the type of HRT you prefer – pills, patches or gel – instead of being restricted to the cheapest form of HRT on the market. If you don't have a computer or are not sure how to search for buying HRT online, then find someone who does.

HRT from the Pharmacist

Before the advent of the NHS when the state became a monopoly provider of health care many people went to the local chemist shop where the pharmacist was trusted to diagnose a range of conditions and dispense medicines. People often preferred to use this service – you didn't have to make an appointment – you could do it with the rest of your shopping and, if you didn't get on with the 'medicine' the pharmacist would recommend something else. This service would be perfect for menopausal women who need to change their prescription from time to time, or try something new.

There is a move in this direction. Pharmacists are now allowed to dispense the morning after pill and statins to reduce heart attacks in men, both of which were previously only available on prescription. At long last the government is considering proposals to enable pharmacists to give advice on whether your symptoms indicate that you have started the menopause, as well as prescribing HRT where appropriate.

Chapter 8
TAKING CHARGE OF YOUR MENOPAUSE

Historical comparisons - A lack of understanding -
Do-it-yourself-kit – Thyroid symptoms -
A cautionary tale of three friends

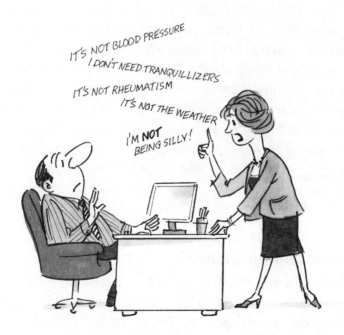

Dear Teresa Gorman,

"I had no menstruation from the age of 28. I thought it odd but I wasn't troubled. I didn't really register it as a malfunction. I thought it only idiosyncratic. Only slowly did I start to become tired, even when I had done nothing and I became increasingly irritable.

My GP eventually picked up my complete lack of periods and recommended HRT - but I had many reservations.

My GP continued to push me towards HRT, but I dithered for more than six months. Eventually I took Premarin and noticed the difference within the first week.

I was becoming an old woman at 30. Now that I am on HRT I have my life back and I have lots of energy and pleasure, too. HRT should not be under a cloud. It should be offered to every woman".

Letter from Margaret H.

Menopause doesn't come with an instruction manual. You don't know when it will begin and no two women have the same experience. Nobody ever teaches women about the menopause – they stumble upon it almost by accident when they begin to experience menopause symptoms and half the time they don't even recognise them. Outside the grim jargon of the medical profession there is no word in the language for menopause other than 'the change', and even that was whispered by one woman to another as if it were something to be ashamed of.

Historical comparisons

The Daily Telegraph recently asked its readers to nominate three inventions which they think have had the biggest influence on our lives. Professor Colin Blakemore, Chief

Executive of the Medical Research Council, nominated the Pill which was not only responsible for sexual liberation and feminism in the 'Swinging Sixties', but also gave young women control of their own body instead of being its slave. But when the Pill was first made available it created uproar which still, to some extent, continues today as shown in a recent attempt to restrict its availability. Similar arguments are now being raised against the use of the Morning After pill.

HRT is even more remarkable because it transforms and extends the active lives of older women in a way that nothing else can. The day will come when HRT will be nominated, not only because it offers older women similar control, but also gives protection against the perils of old age. This won't occur until older women are as valued in society as young women are today and then it, too, will be as highly regarded and as universally popular.

All these medical advances could, and should, be nominated. There has never been a time when *women* were given such an opportunity to decide for *themselves* how to control their biology and, in doing so, are liberated.

A lack of understanding

It is one of the great menopause myths that your mother and grandmother sailed through it. Until recent times most women died before they reached the menopause, worn out with child bearing by the time they were 50. Our generation lives longer, thanks to medical progress and better nutrition, but the quality of the extra years depends largely on how you deal with the menopause.

Some GPs still take the view that the 'change' is not life threatening - but they are wrong. This is not a passing phase but a warning that radical changes are taking place in your body. The obvious signs, such as an end to your periods or hot flushes, pale into insignificance when compared with the internal changes which will become obvious some years later when you develop bone or heart problems. That is why it is vitally important that you understand the changes happening to you and *take charge of the situation.* If your GP is unsympathetic and suggests that you should grin and bare it, ask to be referred to a gynaecologist who specialises in health problems of women.

Some doctors prefer to diagnose a woman by her age and symptoms but this can be very unreliable. Every woman's experience of menopause is different. Even irregular periods are not a completely reliable indication. Some women's periods stop for months and then start again and you could find yourself pregnant having given up on contraception. In these circumstances you need to stop taking HRT until you make your mind up on what you want to do next.

Do-it-yourself test kit

The latest aid to women who want to take charge of their menopause is the 'do-it-yourself' test kit. If your periods are irregular and you regularly have a 'fuzzy head', hot flushes or short-term memory loss then the quickest way to discover whether your oestrogen levels are low and you are in need of hormone replacement, is to find out for yourself.

The kit works like a pregnancy test. You dip a testing strip into a sample of urine and it takes a few minutes to give you a result. Two tests may be needed – one week apart. It indicates whether your symptoms are due to low levels of female hormones and reassures you that your symptoms are not caused by something more serious, such as thyroid deficiency.

Thyroid symptoms

An under active thyroid can cause symptoms similar to those of menopause. An acquaintance of mine was given HRT because her age indicated that her symptoms were probably due to menopause but then her daughter, aged 29, developed similar symptoms. These included tiredness, sweating, nervousness, palpitations, weight loss and hair loss. A simple blood test revealed that she was suffering from thyroid deficiency, and it turned out that this was also the cause of her mother's symptoms. This is a rare coincidence, but if HRT does not solve your 'menopause problems' they may be due to some other cause.

A cautionary tale of three friends

Some women insist that they prefer to let nature takes its course and are prepared to put up with their menopause symptoms. Even personal friends have told me that they were going to grow old gracefully without HRT. I have watched, helpless, as their health deteriorated until they became physical wrecks. Their early signs of menopause – aching back, aches and pains in the joints, were followed by physical and emotional problems, which turned them into invalids. If this is growing old gracefully there is not much joy in it. Several friends have taken different decisions.

Della's tale

Della was a striking-looking woman. You could always pick her out in a crowd by her beautiful head of curly auburn hair. A successful writer and publisher she worked all day long at her computer and helped me to publicise HRT. But when she reached the menopause her doctor discouraged her from using HRT - which was quite common in those days. Now she is paying the price.

After I was elected to Parliament we rarely had time to meet but we kept in touch by telephone. When I retired and wrote a book about my life in Parliament, I naturally invited her to the launch. The room was crowded but I noticed the arrival of an old lady, bent almost double, shuffling along in slippers - on the arm of a young man. I didn't recognise her until I noticed her hair – still curly but snow white.

> *"I know. I should have taken your advice"*, she said, even before I had time to open my mouth. Crippled with osteoporosis and arthritis she could no longer use the computer because of carpel tunnels – erosion of the bones in her fingers. The arches of her feet had dropped too, hence the slippers. She had all the classical symptoms of osteoporosis. *"I didn't bring my stick with me"*, she said. *"I didn't want you to think I was an old lady"*.

Jill's tale

Jill and I were at college together. A country girl, she became the village schoolmistress, married a local farmer, raised two lovely children and kept an eye on her elderly parents. Out in all weathers, doing unmentionable things to sheep's bottoms, in her spare time she raised funds for a local charity.

At 50, she joined me in taking HRT and, like me, she swore by it. And although her mother, aged 70, died of breast cancer she took the decision to continue with HRT. At 70, she too developed a lump in her breast and had it removed and, on the recommendation of her GP, stopped using HRT. She had radiology and Tamoxifen to suppress the possibility of cancer in her other breast. But the hot flushes persisted and became unbearable, so, she was switched to Arimidex. *'Tamoxifen and Arimidex have played hell with me and given me such awful side effects'.* Every joint in her body ached. *'I think it would be easier if I just died!!'.* Now she is thinking about going back to HRT against her GP and Gynaecologist's wishes.

Chemotherapy, with its horrible side effects, only works while you are taking it, so, you will have to put up with the side effects for the rest of your life.

Women are routinely recommended radiotherapy to kill off any cancer cells that may remain and prevent them spreading to other parts of the body. Having tried all these treatments, Jill now shares my opinion that, given the option, she would prefer to have both breasts removed, go back to HRT and get on with her life.

Mary's tale

Mary wrote to me from Australia for advice. She had been using HRT when she was diagnosed with cancer in both breasts and had a double mastectomy.

> *'I didn't feel physically handicapped except for having to come off HRT – which was hellish. I don't feel my health is really optimised without it. When I saw my breast cancer surgeon for a check up and told him I wanted to go back on to it he said he hadn't got a problem with that. But, my gynaecologist disagreed - afraid of being sued, I suspect. I'm still in a kind of limbo. Some of my friends use Livial but even in these cases their doctors are trying to wean them off it for some reason'.*

These are mature and intelligent women and my advice, for what it is worth, is to go back to HRT because the benefits outweigh the risk. Some doctors are over cautious because of the fear of being sued. My view is that women should be allowed to make their own decision. Fortunately, the free market has come to the aid of women who find themselves in this predicament because HRT is available via the Internet (See Chapter 7).

Chapter 9
AM I LOSING MY MIND?

*The change of life - Hormones and personality -
Saving your sanity*

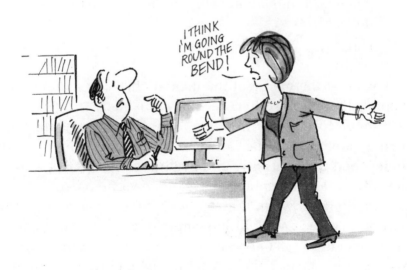

Dear Mrs Gorman,

"I gave up my job which I loved because I seriously thought I was going mad. I was absent-minded and bad-tempered to a frightening degree. I took no pride in my appearance or my house   just sat around crying most of the day. Stephen, my husband, had a horrible time: no kindness, no sex-life. When I went to see my GP he was cruel beyond belief. He just laughed at me and told me to accept that I was getting old. Grudgingly the doctor gave me a hospital referral.

The hospital treated me like a sensible human being and a course of HRT pills was prescribed. After only six weeks life started to feel good again.

I regret that I was pushed out of my job at least five years before I would have chosen. But what is that, so long as you are fit and competent and have a life that is, at best, delightful?"

Letter from Eileen J.

A woman at the mercy of the mental effects of menopause as graphically described by Eileen, is more likely to be dismissed as difficult to get on with rather than someone needing tender loving care. This effect of menopause has been very little understood until recently and even less that HRT can correct the situation. Hormones have a powerful effect on your personality and, when they go haywire, so does your outlook on life. There is very little sympathy amongst colleagues or management – usually male – of the turmoil women experience – at just the same time as men are reaching the peak of their career.

The change of life

When I entered Parliament in 1987, I discovered that the NHS was handing out more prescriptions for tranquillisers than for anything else, most of them prescribed for middle-aged women feeling 'under the weather'. If they suspected that it was something to do with menopause they probably didn't like to mention it to their (usually male) GPs. Much more likely, these women were just not thinking straight because menopause causes mental confusion. Not every GP would have automatically asked the right questions, such as 'are your periods irregular?' and my postbag indicates that some GPs still believe that women are making a fuss about what, to them, seems a natural event.

How women behave and how they think is governed not by the heart but by the brain – which is itself powerfully influenced by hormones. At menopause, when your female hormones are running down, mental confusion and lethargy can be the result. HRT puts your mind back in charge of your body - instead of your body ruling your mind. When I began talking publicly about the menopause I received piles of letters, not only from women but also from family members, saying life at home was impossible because their wife or their mother was 'up in the air' one minute and 'down in the dumps' the next. Personally, you may not be aware that your emotions are in turmoil but those close to you certainly will.

The changes in your behaviour resemble the turmoil that took place at puberty when your hormones were also in turmoil. Then your body was beginning to mature; now it is beginning to grow old! Both events bring about changes in your personality that you are unaware of. But your family and the people you work with will almost certainly notice that there is something different about you. You are much more likely to fall out with people without realising that it is probably your fault. Half the battle is becoming aware of what is happening to you and remedying the situation. It's common to hear women say how much better they feel when they are taking HRT

Hormones and personality

'Why can't a woman be like a man?' asked Professor Higgins in My Fair Lady. The professor was obviously under the influence of testosterone, which turned him into a bully. Eliza, influenced by female hormones, was more inclined to avoid confrontation and try to please the old goat.

The more you know about the effects of your female hormones the more you understand your own behaviour and why women, too, can become extremely violent and aggressive when they have an imbalance of hormones. Most of all you will realise that losing these hormones can lead to a change of personality. For many women hormone replacement is a necessity if they are to continue to lead a normal life.

Do you recognise any of these symptoms? "Where are my keys?" "What did I come upstairs for?" "Has anyone seen my shopping list?" If you are 'becoming forgetful' it is a sign that you are on your way to menopause and in need of HRT.

You may be able to cope at home but at work, when your mind goes blank, it is embarrassing, especially if you are in a roomful of men who are unlikely to be sympathetic much less understand the cause of your discomfort. Don't panic. You are not losing your mind; it's just that your hormones are on the blink and affecting your memory. The brain and hormones work closely together and HRT can re-establish the connection and spare you the embarrassment.

Saving your sanity

Menopause wreaks havoc with women's minds and makes it difficult to concentrate or remember new facts. The stress in women's lives combined with a drop in the hormone, oestrogen, makes them struggle to learn information in the way they did when they were younger. Research shows that many menopausal women also have difficulty recalling faces or names, causing them to worry that their memories are fading.

Remembering was easy when you were young; you were learning new things all the time. But by 50 you have trouble concentrating. By 60 you forget important engagements. By the time you reach 70 you can remember a face but not the name that goes with it and that's when 'old thing-a-ma-bob' becomes your regular chum.

If you reach 80, the chances are you won't remember how to turn on the gas or whether you have turned it off. You may leave the hot water tap running all day. You become a danger to yourself as well as the neighbours and, without someone to keep an eye on you, you may end up in full time care. Early signs of memory loss lead to mental confusion, known as Alzheimer's disease or senile dementia, by the time you reach old age.

Menopause is not a time to sit back and 'let nature take its course'. You need outside activity - keeping in touch with friends and relatives or taking up line dancing, swimming, golf or bowls! Doing crosswords is one of the best ways to keep your mind active.

What about a part time job? B&Q stores are not the only employers who recognise the value of older employees who are more reliable and have more patience with awkward customers. The antidote to old age has not yet been invented but HRT is the best option so far.

Chapter 10
GROWING UP WITH HORMONES

Why boys and girls differ – Battle of the hormones –
Family values - Understanding your daughters

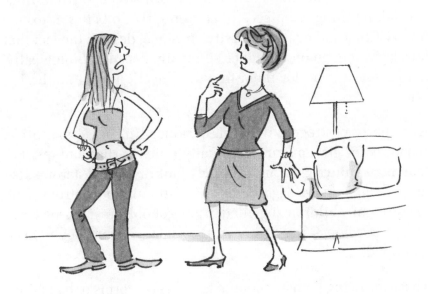

From the moment we are conceived our sex hormones influence every aspect of our being. Even before we are born, they play a key role in the development of the brain and determine the degree of masculinity or femininity in our character. Having spent my early career teaching children I have observed that little girls are more 'sensitive' than boys from the moment they enter school. Having said goodbye to their mothers at the school gates, they usually stand around talking or playing co-operative games, while boys wheel off round the playground shouting and chasing each other or getting into fights. The difference in their behaviour is the result of their hormones.

Why boys and girls differ

Little girls are quicker than boys to learn reading and writing while the boys are much better at exploring their surroundings and taking things to pieces. Later on girls do better at exams up to GCSEs and even university entrance, despite the fact that fewer of them go on to higher education because, biologically, the pressure is on for them to quit education for a mothering role.

At puberty oestrogen, which is produced in large quantities, accounts for girls maturing sexually much earlier and quicker than boys. Boys grow more slowly, but their testosterone also makes them more aggressive and difficult to control. The majority of children expelled from school are teenage boys whose hormones are raging as they change from boyhood to manhood.

These 'growing pains' accounts for extreme forms of behaviour in teenagers - from boredom to self-harm – as the brain learns to adjust.

As an alternative to discipline or punishment, perhaps we should do more by developing hormone therapy for teenagers to help them through this difficult stage in their lives. Uncontrollable behaviour can lead them into serious trouble with authority, including the police, when parents fail to discipline them.

The history of stable societies is predicated on young people being guided by their elders during this impressionable stage in growing up. A disciplined environment in which young people learn to cope with the effect of their hormones is essential. The anti-discipline culture fashionable today is diametrically opposed to their needs in coping with powerful biological changes.

Speaking as a biologist, the need to discipline young people is not unique; it exists amongst all other groups of mammals. What is unique is that, today, we ignore the need to discipline the young at the very time in their life when they are most in need of a firm and guiding hand.

Battle of the hormones

Thanks to contraception this is the first generation of women who have a choice on when to start a family and many women put it off while developing their career. But some women who delay having their children until they are over 30 may never conceive. Their only option is IVF and anyone who has tried it would tell you that it is physically and emotionally draining and may empty your bank balance.

A late baby will be a teenager just when you enter your menopause stage and both of you will be at the mercy of your hormones when their hormones are hyperactive and yours are draining away. This is a recipe for family strife.

You may be feeling like hell just as they become difficult to handle and family life becomes impossible. You find yourself arguing about whether they can have a boyfriend or girlfriend to stay overnight while they think you are being unreasonable. Rivalry and resentment festers on both sides - made worse by the clash of hormones – although neither of you are aware of it. The last thing both of you need is friction.

Family values

As menopause approaches, your family may also notice changes in your behaviour. One minute you are 'nice old mum', the next you lose your temper and yell at them. Some women I know – including my own mother – take to throwing crockery at their spouse.

"What am I supposed to have done now?" cry members of the family. You may not realise it but your emotions are in turmoil. This is the time when your partner decides to stop over at the club or the pub for a few drinks with the lads to delay the inevitable rows when he gets home. What on earth can you do about it?

There is an intimate connection between hormones and the brain and in the rundown to menopause it begins to receive irregular signals from your body. Like an electric circuit with a fault in it, it switches your moods on and off. Menopause is a time of mental as well as physical confusion, which can end in divorce. It creates problems at work as well as at home. HRT benefits not only the women who use it, but their families and their workmates as well.

If menopause starts early there is nothing you can do to stop it. You cannot turn back the clock to prolong your 'fertile' life. If your mother or other close female relatives had an early menopause it may happen to you. This can be a problem for women who delay starting a family because of their career.

Nature has designed women for having children while they are young – starting in their teens. There is no guarantee that you will remain fertile until you are 50.

Understanding your daughters

Conflicts, which arise between mothers and daughters, have more to do with hormones than stubbornness. Teenage daughters may develop extreme forms of behaviour whilst learning to cope with the ups and downs of their hormones, particularly before a period when levels of both female hormones plummet. Their behaviour at this time of the month, referred to as pre-menstrual tension - or PMT - can spill over into self-harm. Hormone therapy can restore normal behaviour in teenagers, but is often overlooked by busy GPs who are not trained to deal with personality problems.

Under the French penal code pre-menstrual tension is classified as 'temporary insanity' and is accepted as a legitimate defence in criminal cases. In Britain the pre-menstrual tension defence has twice been accepted in reducing a murder charge to manslaughter. As a Member of Parliament I visited women prisoners convicted of murdering their partner. Having heard the circumstances I was convinced that some of them should have been offered a retrial because they had suffered enough physical abuse already. But I have yet to meet a Home Secretary – almost always a man - who was ready to give them the benefit of the doubt.

Amongst women prisoners, suicides, violence and dangerous behaviour are also markedly higher at the time of PMT. Behavioural changes, which happen during this phase of the menstrual cycle and PMT (pre-menstrual tension) should not be looked upon as a minor nuisance. Criminal actions could be prevented if hormone replacement were offered.

These days the empty nest syndrome is becoming something of a fantasy. Teenage children just don't move away from home in the way they used to.

Student offspring cling on through university years. Or worse still, decide to move back home when they have finished studying. They claim they can't afford a place of their own. In my day you were expected to find 'lodgings' in someone else's house while the parents were free to enjoy growing old together. Today's parents are not 'old' at 50 – they may be out playing golf – or learning to.

HRT won't solve these family problems but it will help you to keep a cool head and make them easier to bear!

Chapter 11
MOVIES, SOAPS AND BBC PRIME TIME

Breasts and bottoms - The Movies – TV Soaps -
The Archers – BBC Prime time – A historical view

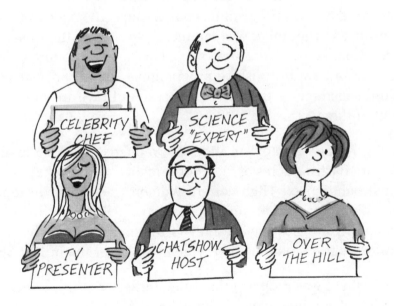

If TV and radio don't have as many middle-aged women presenters as middle-aged men, what message are they sending out to their viewers and listeners? The BBC is one of the most chauvinistic institutions in the Country. Where, in the world of entertainment, are the role models for middle-aged women? The BBC motto is 'Nation Shall Speak Peace Unto Nation' - so long as men do most of the talking. It certainly doesn't live up to its mandate to represent all of the people all of the time because middle-aged women are virtually excluded after the nine o'clock watershed hour. This is all the more surprising when the BBC's Directors of television, radio and music, are middle-aged women who are in a position to correct this anomaly.

It is not as if there is a shortage of jobs. Television is dominated by middle-aged men who not only present mainstream news programmes but are also given a second job fronting entertainment programmes - topping up their pension pots. Chat shows, quiz shows, cookery and gardening shows, ancient and natural history programmes, are all presented by middle-aged men – the same old faces - until we are sick of the sight of them.

Young women do appear after the watershed hour so long as they are flashing acres of flesh presumably because they attract a male audience. High calibre women presenters disappear from our screens at around eight o'clock. By excluding older women from hosting late evening chat shows the BBC reinforces the prejudice that women are 'over the hill' at 50.

If ever there was a subject that in real life is almost exclusively the lot of women it is cooking for the family. But on TV frenetic young men and foul-mouthed Glaswegians who splutter all over the food whilst throwing their weight about dominate it. Where are the successors to the 'Two Fat Ladies' and Delia Smith, loved and admired by women for their sensible tips and friendly banter, always remembering to point out the little details which women need to know to make a success of their recipes?

Breasts and bottoms

Of course, breasts are not the only part of our anatomy used to draw attention – mainly male attention – to a product or cause. Hips and bottoms, too, are potent sex symbols, hugely attractive to men who subconsciously size them up as a sign of fertility and the ability of a woman to produce their offspring.

Such is the power of these symbols that highly trained plastic surgeons will, for a handsome fee, implant plastic sacks filled with silicone to enlarge the breasts or give your bottom a 'lift'. You have only to catch a glimpse of grotesquely deformed young women on TV shows to see what powerful signals they convey.

Nor is this a recent phenomenon. There have been many periods throughout history when young women enhanced their chance of marriage by displaying their cleavage – or 'putting their puddings out for treacle' – as my mother used to say.

Long before the bra was invented, young women in Regency times (in search of a husband) propped up their breasts so that their cleavage sat provocatively above the line of the dress. French women were even more risqué. During Napoleon's reign they exposed one breast, usually with a ring pierced through the nipple.

Edwardian women went one step further by inventing the bustle to enhance their bottoms as well. Anyone who watches television will know that women's bottoms are used to draw attention to a rather squatty-botty car. Today, anyone travelling on London's underground has a reasonable chance of viewing more of a woman's bottom than they bargained for – especially if they are behind them on the escalator. The biggest selling poster produced by Athena shows a woman tennis player baring her bottom – even Wimbledon has joined the bandwagon.

The Movies

Today, the whole fantasy world of the movies, which holds up a mirror to human behaviour, cuts older women out of its scripts. Producers ruthlessly exclude women over 40 from the more glamorous roles as romantic heroines unless, of course, they have swapped the casting couch for plastic surgery. Their worth is judged by their looks. Hollywood makes women feel ashamed to say how old they are, while young women are chased across the screen by old men in their dotage. Men don't age in the movies - they become more distinguished.

Does this matter? Well, yes it does, because every woman in the audience will experience menopause and it would be nice if they could relate their symptoms to that of their movie heroines as a normal part of a woman's experience instead of something to hide. Film directors, like most men, are staggeringly ill-informed about 'female problems' so it's not surprising that they run a mile from a film star on the set who had to pause for a short break while having a hot flush. But some filmmakers are beginning to reflect a change in attitude towards older women. The *Graduate* featured Mrs. Robinson, an older woman playing a younger man for sex. *Shirley Valentine* was in a loveless marriage when she found romance on a Greek island with a boatman that she picked up on holiday. An in *Calendar Girls* a whole bunch of middle-class, middle-aged women took their kit off for charity.

Perhaps a sequel to *Calendar Girls* could be *Menopause Matrons*. Not much of a title, but it could be one hell of a funny movie and break a taboo. The plot could revolve around the husbands who would almost certainly die first leaving our heroines to go on surfboarding into the sunset with a packet of HRT pills in their pockets.

TV Soaps

Week after week, the scriptwriters scratch their heads for a new angle to keep the audience numbers up. They claim the programmes are a slice of real life. Well, so is the menopause. Times have changed and the Soaps are out of date. Women are no longer over the hill at 50.

Teenage illegitimacy, young men kissing one another, attempted incest, depression and schizophrenia can all be found in the Soaps. But the middle-aged women are all weary characters - left to struggle on through menopause problems which may be alluded to but are never actually featured as part of the plot. 'Middle-aged women's problems' are considered to be too sensitive for family viewing.

The Archers

After all the missed opportunities for the soaps to tackle the subject of HRT, it has been left to the good old Archers to do a bit of groundbreaking. After years when the script slavishly followed Ministry of Agriculture press handouts, it has temporarily abandoned organic vegetables for Cathy's hot flushes for which HRT 'cake', made from vegetables, was recommended as a cure, a subtle plug for organic solutions to menopause problems. It gave the scriptwriters a golden opportunity to explain menopause in ponderous language.

Vegetable remedies will not cure hot flushes but they could spawn a new rural industry to replace the broiler chickens, sheep and cows who lost their lives in the greatest soap opera of them all, written by the Ministry of Agriculture Fisheries and Food.

BBC Prime Time

This is where the male ego gets into its stride. Imagine you were on the selection panel interviewing a number of middle-aged candidates for the top job. The men will be 'mature', 'distinguished' by a touch of grey at the temples and the 'character' lines on their face. Women's character lines, called wrinkles, will give the impression of being too old for the job anyway. Yet, a woman's voice is acknowledged to be more soothing and reassuring than a man – and that's why women were used for the speaking clock on the telephone and in-car navigational systems (Sat Nav).

Why is it that greying, middle-aged men always get the top jobs of presenting the News during prime-time television, accompanied by a much younger and prettier woman who reads the 'soft news' stories, leaving the weightier matters to be dealt with by the men.

We are moving into a 'menopause society' where older women will soon predominate but, as newsreaders and presenters, they are still relegated to less popular times or in a subordinate role. These women are all class acts but bottom of the 'A' list when it comes to regular appearances on prime time TV.

The men who control both BBC and ITV are, of course, reflecting their own image and reinforcing the stereotype of men in charge while older women are relegated to a subordinate role. What ever happened to equal opportunities?

A historical view

Throughout history post-menopausal women are depicted in an unfavourable light. The image of the witch was an unmarried, middle-aged woman forced to the fringes of society where she scraped a living as best she could as a midwife or by casting spells for a few groats. Witches were frequently blamed when disasters befell the community and even sacrificed by being burned at the stake. Shakespeare describes the witches in MacBeth as bent double and causing trouble which today would be recognised as osteoporosis.

Our attitude to age is shaped for us in childhood with fairy tales featuring the wicked stepmother, as in Cinderella and Snow White, and the old hag in Hansel and Gretel. They could have been recast as the fairy godmother if only they had access to HRT. Today, post-menopausal women are more likely to be found in a bikini on the beach being ogled by men half their age.

The mad wife locked in the attic in Jane Eyre may well have been the victim of an early menopause. It is not uncommon for women suffering from mental confusion to be thought of as 'going mad'. The brain and hormones work closely together and the mind is sometimes overwhelmed and unable to cope. I don't suppose that Charlotte Bronte had this in mind when she wrote her classic novel but reading between the lines the whole plot smacks of hormone-related sexual frustration leading to the ultimate cruelty of being locked away for life.

Victorian women swooned or had the vapours - classic menopause symptoms. The chaise longue could have been designed for women who needed to put their feet up while they recovered from palpitations or a hot flush. Women consoled themselves with smelling salts but when their pain and suffering became too hard to bear, they took laudanum (opium) then freely available. Queen Victoria herself used laudanum regularly.

Dr. Collis Brown's Linctus, the most popular remedy for the working woman in Victorian times, also contained laudanum. 'Gin palaces', too, were known as their haunts, somewhere to drown their 'sorrows'. That is, if they lived long enough to experience them. Victorian charities like the Salvation Army, crusaded against gin and fallen women, offering religion as an alternative.

Today's breast cancer charities continue the tradition by crusading against women and HRT. So, nothing much has changed then! If the latest planet to be discovered were to be named after a woman that would be real progress because, with the exception of Venus, all the rest have been named after men.

Chapter 12
THE BEAUTY BUSINESS

The cosmetics industry – Skin deep -
Collagen – Hair – Teeth – The mating market -
Keeping up appearances -

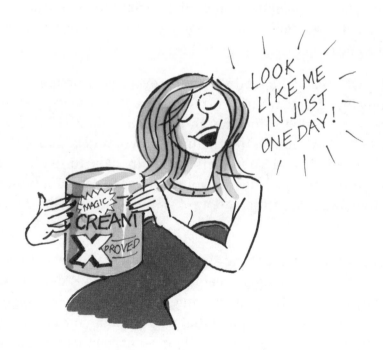

The cosmetics industry

When Estée Lauder died in her nineties in April 2004, the cosmetic business she founded was worth $10 billion, a tribute to the powers of persuasion, coupled with women's insecurity, as their wrinkles begin to show and they lose confidence in their appearance. The signs of ageing in men enhance their opportunities in presenting prime time programmes because wrinkles and greying hair apparently make them look distinguished, endowing them with wisdom and increased earning power. For women, the opposite is true. Young women publicly decry the use of collagen therapy, hormone replacement and other miracles of modern anti-ageing, preferring herbal teas or ridiculously expensive face creams which supposedly contain some new and secret ingredient. Cosmetic companies make their millions by playing on women's fear of ageing and dissatisfaction with their appearance.

In the UK, women spend £5 billion every year on creams and lotions but if you want to make the most of your appearance without spending a fortune on cosmetics, then HRT is your best bet. It stimulates the natural growth and repair of your skin, your hair and your nails and helps you to retain many other attractive qualities of your younger years, including a positive outlook on life and a refusal to grow old – gracefully or otherwise.

The only miraculous thing about cosmetics is the way they are advertised. The claims dreamed up by their PR departments are beyond parody. Advertising agencies must be laughing their heads off at the thought that women believe what they are told. In your 20s you don't really need cosmetics because you are awash with natural oestrogen which revitalises your skin.

In your 30s you are probably bringing up a family – and can't afford pots of expensive creams. And in your 50s they are a waste of money - HRT can do the job for you at a fraction of the price.

The cosmetics industry plays on women's fear of ageing in just the same way as charities play on their horror of developing breast cancer. Both industries are prepared to stretch the truth to gain publicity. Two of L'Oreal's TV adverts were recently banned by the Advertising Standards Authority for wrongly claiming that two of its anti-cellulite creams destroyed fat below the surface of the skin – when skin was designed to protect the underlying layers and to keep things out.

Skin deep

Your skin is not a piece of blotting paper soaking up the latest cream or lotion on offer. You only need soap and water to take off the dirt and a light coating of oil to prevent excessive evaporation of the natural moisture under the skin. It is a waterproof jacket, designed by Nature to protect you from the bugs and dirt. When you see advertisements for cosmetics that promise to 'feed' the underlying layers, take it with a large pinch of salt. If substances could find their way through as easily as that don't you think that every bug, every fungus which lands on the surface, would long since have found a way in? There are more than 10 million bacteria on a square centimetre of human skin but there are very few ways to get in unless your skin is broken, cut or damaged.

You *can* have a good guess at a woman's age by the quality of her skin. It is the first thing people notice when you meet and it sends subliminal signals about your age and general health.

But after menopause, your skin begins to age rapidly as the blood supply beneath the surface of the skin is reduced. Less nourishment reaches the underlying layers, which keep the skin smooth, pink and healthy. You can fill in the fine lines with makeup and add a little colour to the cheeks - but it comes off in the wash.

Your skin is the largest sense organ of your body – about six square metres of it – and a mass of highly sensitive, touchy-feely nerve endings which, although you may not have given the matter much thought, the massage parlour industry thrives on. Their busiest time is the lunch hour when stressed city gents prefer it to a visit to the pub or a coffee and sandwich. And women, too, enjoy their 'me' time in the guise of aromatherapy, complete with incense candles and fragrant oils which make body massage more respectable. I think it's a shame that people have to go to such lengths to enjoy the pleasurable sensations that your skin has to offer.

Collagen

Collagen is the rubbery substance which pads out the underlying layer of your skin to keep it smooth and oestrogen is essential for its production. At menopause, as oestrogen levels fall, the collagen layer collapses and wrinkles begin to appear, followed by sagging cheeks, bags under the eyes and, finally, the dreaded 'turkey neck'. Lines from your nose to the corner of your mouth and from your mouth down to your chin are a sure sign of a lack of collagen beneath the skin. And collagen is not just about wrinkles. It also strengthens your hair, nails and bones. The only thing that will save you from these horrors is maintaining your supply of oestrogen by using HRT and there is no reason ever to give it up.

Hair

Your hair is also an important part of sexual attraction. But even the most fashionable hairdresser cannot make a silk purse out of a sow's ear. Thinning hair is another of the dreaded signs of middle age. It's not that you mind so much about approaching your 60s but approaching your 60s and going bald is

a terrible prospect. Better by far is to stop it from falling out in the first place. Enter our old friend oestrogen, which nurtures the hair roots and continues the cycle of growth and replacement just as it did when you were younger. Whatever your age it is a sure sign that you are still firing on all cylinders and undoubtedly affects the way other people react to you.

Teeth

We British are really good at bad teeth. Next time you look in the mirror don't just criticise the shape of your nose or your wrinkles. Take a good look at your teeth then take out a bank loan, if necessary, to fix them. You can spend a small fortune on cosmetics, or even cosmetic surgery, but nothing does more for your prospects than a really lovely smile and full set of gleaming white teeth.

With age, your gums begin to shrink to reveal little yellow stumps at the roots and eventually your teeth will fall out unless you keep your bones in good condition. The alternative may be a set of dentures to remove each night and put in a pot at your bedside. Is this something you and your partner look forward to? Or have you given up on romance?

The Mating Market

In case you think I am exaggerating the effect of appearance on the opposite sex, a recent study, led by Dr. Craig Roberts at the University of Newcastle, makes fascinating reading:

> *"When a young woman is at her most fertile her scent will change, her skin will glow and look smoother than usual, her lips look more luscious, her hair shinier and eyes more inviting. These signals have evolved as a way to help women capture men's attention. And they are all down to our female hormones – which disappear at menopause. At this time in her cycle, when the probability of conception is highest, she will exude a provocative allure that makes her more attractive to men. She is sending out the message that she is in the 'mating market' and this will be picked up by men who are looking for a long-term partner".*

Leaving aside the flowery prose, without oestrogen, older women do develop masculine characteristics, including hairs in unwanted places. In the absence of their female hormones the residual amount of testosterone which the body continues to make into old age, takes over. It is a fact that, as women grow older their features coarsen and they begin to look more like men. If you don't want to risk this happening to you, then HRT may be the only answer.

Not for nothing do cosmetic ads consistently use smooth-skinned young women to advertise products aimed at middle-aged women desperate to recover that 'inner glow' which, according to Dr. Roberts, makes them so attractive to the opposite sex. But, sexual attraction is not just about appearance; it is also about attitude - which probably accounts for the fact that more and more young men are attracted to older women - and my guess is that HRT may have more than a little to do with it!

Keeping up appearances

Never underestimate the psychological effect of looking good and feeling fit. Going through the menopause can have a depressing effect on your attitude to life. You feel that you are getting old, life's over, so why bother to look nice if no one is going to look at you anyway? But the less trouble you take, the worse you look and the more your fears are realised. Who wants to strike up a conversation with someone who looks weary and worn who hasn't bothered much with how she looks? But HRT will change your outlook on life and if you don't know what to replace those dreary, baggy old clothes with - and you haven't got a hot-line to Trinny and Susannah - 'phone a friend' and take her shopping with you to get an honest opinion. Otherwise, you may end up taking it to the charity shop.

You may no longer be young in years but that doesn't mean you have to give in without a fight. You don't have to pretend you are still a teenager but pampering yourself can lift your spirits and give you a new zest for life. First impressions count. A smart, confident, attractive woman will never be overlooked and ignored. If your partner feels threatened by the 'new' you because he is afraid other men will be attracted to you do not be tempted to fade back into the wallpaper.

Chapter 13
A NEW LEASE OF LIFE

Sex after menopause - Marilyn Monroe and the secret tapes - Lonely hearts column - The Saga saga – Growing old disgracefully – Living alone – Hang on to your houses

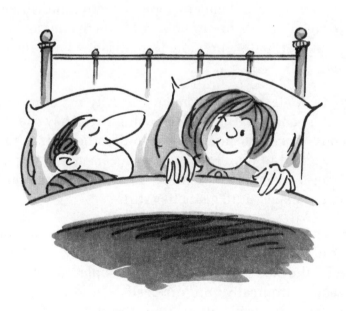

Dear Teresa Gorman,

After my divorce I found myself forced out of the life of a housewife to fend for the family. At first, I made do with routine jobs, which I found very tiring until my doctor put me on to HRT for 'the change'. As my confidence increased I took a course at university and discovered I had a brain. If my husband hadn't left me I'd still be at home doing what I'd always done, only by now I'd be looking after the grandchildren as well. Now I am a professional with a good salary and I love it. I feel as if I've been born again. Hooray for HRT.

Letter from Ann P.

Ann's letter expresses better than I could the remarkable effects which HRT can have on your confidence in circumstances when your life seems to be falling to pieces. It made her stronger and able to cope in a situation which could easily have got the better of her. HRT uncovered an ability in her which she hadn't previously realised – and transformed her life.

Thanks to contraception women over fifty need no longer be worn out by childbearing and, by using HRT, they can improve their confidence and their energy to do other things that they always wanted to do. There has never been a better time for middle-aged women to achieve their full potential and I confidently expect it to get better still.

In the past, women regarded menopause as a liberation from the fear of an unwanted pregnancy. But today - with that fear removed - they are free to experience the pleasure of sex for its own sake. Ironically, middle-aged men lose their sexual potency and, in desperation, they resort to artificial means, including Viagra, to keep their spirits up.

Sex after menopause

At menopause you may feel you are losing your appeal, that you're old and that your partner no longer seems to notice you. After years of living together, it is so easy to take each other for granted. He, too, may start doubting his sexual appeal to women and go out of his way to chat up younger women to prove that he still hasn't 'lost it'.

When the psychological and the outward physical signs of ageing combine, both partners begin to lose self-confidence. HRT can prevent these and similar worries by keeping your interest in a physical relationship alive.

A married woman under extreme stress will reach out and hold her husband's hand and feel immediate relief. The soothing effect of the touch can be seen in scans of areas in the brain that are involved in registering emotional and physical alarm. Women receive significantly more relief from their husbands' touch than from a stranger. This helps to explain one of the longest standing puzzles in social science; why married men and women are healthier on average than their peers. Easy access to an affectionate touch – a hug, a back rub or more – is a very good thing and deeply soothing.

Marilyn Monroe and the secret tapes

In secret tapes of conversations between Marilyn Monroe and her psychologist she revealed that she had never had an orgasm. *"I well remember you said an orgasm happens in the mind and not in the genitals"*, she says. It may well be that the ultra-feminine symbol of our age didn't really have those intimate relationships with the Kennedys – or if she did she was faking it like many women do. If you have been brought up to feel guilty about sex it is jolly difficult to enjoy it. But that doesn't mean you need to give up trying. It would be a shame to miss out on one of life's greatest pleasures.

Lonely Hearts column

The personal adverts in newspapers and magazines offer a near perfect insight into what men seek in women – which is always age-related. The Financial Times often hints at the bonding of hearts by sharing balance sheets. Farmer's Weekly reveals a woman must show dexterity in plucking chickens with extra marks for tractor knowledge. The men can be measured by their acres. Private Eye readers are even more confused in their ambitions.

> *"Serious minded guy, 60s, likes music, theatre, books and outdoors, seeks F, 40s, for mutual benefits".*
>
> *"Recycled bachelor, 50s, n/s, caring, educated, loves countryside, broadminded, seeks younger female".*
>
> *"Anarchistic vegan, 56, eclectic tastes, WLTM, sophisticated F, ideally 30s to enjoy concerts etc. Dislikes TV and religion".*

One well-defined strand is that the male advertisers often seek women twenty or more years younger. Men perceive younger women not just as more attractive but also of greater utility. When you see a beautiful young woman on the arm of a much older man it tells you more about his bank balance than his sexual attraction. Women have always been made to feel self conscious about their age but, no longer. The tables are turning and every other day we read in the Press of a middle-aged woman celebrity marrying a much younger man and I know for a fact that some of them are devotees of HRT.

The very idea of sexual relationships between an older woman and a younger man was treated with derision in most countries, but not in France. The French author, Colette, makes it clear in her novels that a relationship between a younger man and an older woman is nothing out of the ordinary. It helps younger men to learn the art of giving sexual pleasure which makes them better husbands when they decide to marry – and a similar theme was portrayed in the movie, *The Graduate*.

Today, women need not be marginalized because of their age and hormone replacement plays a key role in this change in attitude. Women need no longer accept that they are over-the-hill at 50.

The Saga saga

Saga – the fastest growing travel agents in the business - reports a boom in holiday breaks for the over 50s to far-flung destinations paid for by re-mortgaging the family home. Safari trips, visits to Antarctica, scuba diving, white water rafting and trekking in Peru and Borneo – all activities once confined to their sons and daughters - are coming up fast while the younger generation stays at home working to pay towards their college fees. As more of us live into old age it will cause problems for the government – big financial problems – so planning now for how fit you will be in your 80s or 90s is essential if you don't want to become a burden to your children or grandchildren and, worse still, dependent on the state.

When I returned from teaching in the United Sates, my local school Inspector offered me 'a nice little job as a deputy head'. The thought of going back to where I left off did not appeal. I was 40ish, already using HRT which gave me the energy to set up in business and the gamble paid off. Next, I was elected to

Westminster City Council for a seat which no-one, including me, expected to win and I went on to be elected to Parliament, at the age of 57, the oldest woman ever to be a first time M.P. None of this was planned and I believe that HRT gave me the confidence and the energy to carry it through. Politics is a twenty-four hour a day job and you need to have all your wits about you. HRT never let me down. In the male-dominated world of business and politics women need that extra dimension of self-confidence to compete with their testosterone-fuelled male colleagues.

Growing old disgracefully

Natural selection did not take into account that twentieth century women may not be willing to retreat from the scene and prepare to die. Marriage records show an increased trend for older women to marry younger men.

Fortified by HRT, with a dab or two of testosterone, they can keep up with a young suitor half their age. Joan Collins is a great role model for HRT users. Just try telling her to come off it because of the latest scare story. She has made it clear that, come what may, she intends to stick with it. Good for her. And long may she retain the ability to keep up with the gorgeous Percy. Why should men have all the fun!

The whole attitude to sexual relationships has undergone a sea change over the past three decades and, whereas younger women today are more relaxed about sex, the majority of older women still carry the burden of inhibitions related to society's disapproval in the past of promiscuous behaviour on the part of women. Men, of course, have always had their sins forgiven. Women who have experienced sexual difficulties in the past use their advancing years as an excuse to avoid sex altogether. Which is a pity because nature designed lovemaking to be irresistibly enjoyable – even if it only lasts a few minutes!

Divorced wives used to get the thin end of the wedge both financially and with little hope of finding a new partner. But the latest report from the Office of National Statistics points out that one in four marriages now involve an older woman and a younger man – a complete reversal of the situation which used to apply. These modern day marriages are turning the tables on the whole of human history and must surely contain an interest in sex to keep up with their younger partners. HRT helps you to take a much more relaxed attitude to sex – even solo sex – and makes you less frigid.

Living alone

A report from the Office of National Statistics on population trends paints a gloomy picture in which half the women over 75 are living alone and warns that this number is set to rise dramatically. The government views old age in negative terms. Women over 50 outnumber men in the population by 1.5million which accounts for the fact that they are cluttering up our old people's homes. The government thinks that the only way to cope with this demographic imbalance is to build more care homes, ignoring the fact that HRT enables women to be more active, involved and independent.

As older women become more financially independent and self-confident there is no reason why they shouldn't enjoy living alone and treasure independence and privacy. Men might want to be married for a variety of reasons, most of which involve them being waited on, and that is one of the reasons why they take on a younger wife.

Hang onto your houses

The British state pension is amongst the lowest in the western world and is dependent on future generations of taxpayers to provide for older people. When company pensions go pear shaped you can find yourself in financial difficulties and the government can't be trusted not to pillage your private pension fund.

Your house is the best bet for income in your old age, so don't make it over to the children too soon. You can't expect your children to be willing to look after you in your old age. And would they need to if 'the oldies' were still able to look after themselves? By using HRT you can stay independent longer.

Chapter 14

OVERCOMING OLD AGE WITH HRT

Seventy plus – what lies ahead of us? -
Sir John Peel - Margaret Thatcher – Wendy Cooper -
Fay Weldon – Barbara Cartland

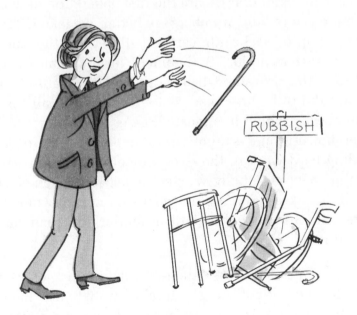

Dear Teresa Gorman,

I'm not sure how I heard about HRT. I recall an item on 'Women's Hour' but I had heard about it before then. So, I did a search on the PC at our local library and then asked our GP for her advice. She wasn't opposed to it but had so many qualifications it sounded like a rejection. I remember we laughed when I said that I'd heard that the Queen Mother's long life and energy was an advert for HRT. She joked it was probably more likely gin. I asked her to look up what her medical journals had to say about HRT – then we both agreed to try it out. We've never looked back.

Letter from Linda N.

Seventy plus – what lies ahead of us?

It is easy to forget that we are the first generation of women to reach old age in large numbers – whether we take HRT or not. Greatly improved health care at all levels, the control of diseases such as polio, TB, rheumatic fever and measles. Birth control – the unwanted babies and infant deaths in an age without the pill. Improved diet – yes, despite all the furore about obesity which in almost all cases is in your own hands. Better housing and sanitation. All these went to ease the grinding hard work of the lives women used to lead without washing machines, hoovers, electric kettles – even electricity. For all the jokes about coal in the bath, for most women it was a life without much fun and a shorter life than has been granted to us.

So for goodness sake let's celebrate what is being offered. You hear a lot about it not being 'natural' to want to feel and behave in your seventies as you did in your fifties and sixties. OK, perhaps Mother Nature never expected you to live this long.

She switches off the very hormones which keep you attractive and active, closing down the very hormones that keep you mentally alert, sexually and physically active, and interested in the world around you. But then, this is the very same Mother Nature that would have had you dead from diphtheria by the age of three. What sort of mother is that?

Sir John Peel

People 'in the know' have benefited from HRT for longer than you may think. Sir John Peel, gynaecologist to the Queen Mother, pioneered HRT in this country and had this to say about it.

> *"I am convinced from experience that Hormone Replacement Therapy can be of immense help to a great number of women. This book should do much to educate women about themselves and stimulate them to seek medical advice instead of putting up with unpleasant and at times disastrous symptoms in the belief that they are the inevitable consequences of being a woman who must grin and bear it all".* Introduction to No Change by Wendy Cooper.

The Queen Mother's lively mind and sense of humour which accompanied her to the end of her active and colourful life, is typical of older women who have used HRT. I would like to think that she, too, benefited from one of the greatest advances in women's healthcare.

Margaret Thatcher

When, in 1987, I unexpectedly joined the ranks of Conservative candidates, I was interviewed by journalist, Peter McKay. For want of something better to write about a new face on the political scene, he dubbed me the 'Queen of HRT' then went on to speculate whether it accounted for Margaret Thatcher's phenomenal energy. Maybe we wouldn't be having this debate if it had been publicly known that she was benefiting from HRT - especially as most women of 'her age' were drawing their pension. I had my suspicions that HRT had something to do with her boundless energy – she was rumoured to need only four hours of sleep a night! I didn't do much to deny the possibility but I dared not ask Margaret if it were true. She was, after all, the Prime Minister and I was a new recruit.

It was not until after she left office, when she invited me for tea and biscuits at her home that I summoned up the courage to ask her whether my suspicion was correct.

"Yes, dear, I have a patch," she said and she tapped her hip as if to indicate that the patch was in place. At that moment Margaret joined the ranks of my HRT heroines – alongside the Queen Mother - and a myriad of high-powered women most of who have yet to 'come out' and admit that it is the source of their attraction and superhuman energy. HRT has come a long way since those early days in the 1980s when the Amarant Trust was formed to break through the ignorance about HRT in this country.

Wendy Cooper

Wendy Cooper, who pioneered the use of HRT on this side of the Atlantic, is now in her late 70s and goes surfing each day alongside hordes of young people a quarter of her age. Fit as a fiddle and bright as a button, she attributes her active lifestyle to HRT and what it can do for the quality of life in later years. Wendy says it is nonsense to suggest that there is some arbitrary length of time for taking HRT and in the USA, where HRT has been available since the 1940s, women in their 80s are more likely to be found exercising on the beach or on the golf course than languishing in a residential care home.

Fay Weldon

Fay Weldon, novelist, playwright and screenwriter is a great fan of HRT and swears that it has also kept her own writing career afloat.

She told me the story of her mother, also a writer in her younger years, who, at the age of seventy, needed full time care because it was unsafe for her to live alone. Oblivious of her surroundings, rocking backwards and forwards in her chair, she barely recognised her own daughter when she visited. In despair at her mother's hopeless condition, Fay persuaded the doctor to prescribe HRT. The results were amazing.

"It was like a miracle. My mother began to regain her memory and her personality. She became a person again". Fay told me.

She was able to leave the nursing home and live independently. She even took up writing again. Sadly, as a result of this latest scare, at the age of 93 she was taken off HRT on the grounds that she had been taking it too long and might get cancer! Within the year she fell into a depression and died. *"Doctors are quite mad"*, said Fay.

Barbara Cartland

Dame Barbara, famous author of hundreds of love stories, first wrote about HRT in the 1960's, long before it became generally known in the UK. I first met her at the House of Commons when she was already well into her 80's. You couldn't possibly miss her in the crowded Central Lobby - dressed to death in pink from top to toe.

"I went on natural oestrogen myself after I had a hysterectomy and felt just wonderful on it. My daughter, the Countess of Dartmouth, went on it in her mid-forties as preventative medicine, and my mother was put on it at the age of 96, by her doctor to protect against risk of further fractures. So that was three generations of us all on HRT.

I'm now eighty-eight and I could not be without my HRT. It makes all the difference to my feeling of well-being, my health and fitness. I also find, as do many of the women who write to me, that it helps to keep our skin soft and supple as well as making all the difference to our love lives. The benefits are spectacular", Barbara told me as we chatted over tea on the Terrace.

She confided to me that she had recently fallen on a concrete floor in her local supermarket - and hadn't even chipped a bone! I don't know what surprised me the most, the image of Barbara pushing a supermarket trolley wearing one of her feather-decked hats, or spread-eagled on the floor in an exotic pink dress. I last saw her shortly before she died. She was still upright and glamorous, enjoying every moment.

In my travels I have met women doctors, lawyers and university professors still practicing their professions in their 80s and 90s who attribute their health and mental alertness to HRT. There are other clinical studies which prove that some of the worst nightmares of old age can be avoided or even reversed with the use of hormone replacement.

With the exception of Joan Collins, few women in the public eye like to talk about their age - or the fact that they are using

HRT except, of course, when they are still active and seen as a phenomenon – like the Queen Mother. In the 1940s, the author, Wendy Cooper, was recommending HRT in her classic book *"No Change"*. She still regularly body surfs off the Gower coast with surfers in their teens and twenties. The author Fay Weldon tells a story of her mother who enjoyed her independence in her eighties and nineties until the doctors stopped her HRT. And, of course, there is no stopping Margaret Thatcher. The latest government 'wheeze' is to give us an MOT at different intervals in our life but older women wouldn't need one if they had been encouraged to use HRT from the moment their natural supply of hormones runs out at menopause.

Chapter 15

INTERNATIONAL AND NATIONAL STUDIES

The Japanese Study – The American Study – The British Study – What the rest of the world has to say about HRT

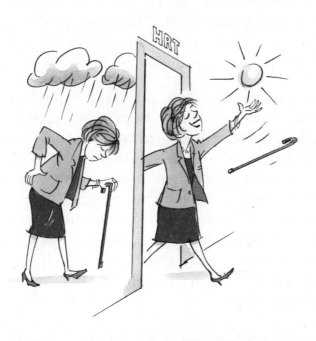

Studies in many countries have demonstrated that HRT can improve the quality of life for women in care who have already succumbed to the devastating effects of senility.

The Japanese Study

In Japan the National Mental Health conducted a study of very old patients in which women with dementia were given HRT treatment over a six-week period to see whether it could improve their mental condition. The trials were conducted under scrupulous scientific conditions and were reported in the Proceedings of the International Congress on the Menopause 1993.

The Report states that, remarkably, the patients showed significant improvement in recent as well as long-term memory. Their personality related to their mood. Their sleeping and feeding habits were much better. The effects of the treatment were similar to those seen when patients were given anti-depressant pills. These improvements were not only noted by the doctors conducting the tests but also by the nurses and patients' families.

> "These improvements, especially in memory and mood, are the same as those frequently reported in younger, post-menopausal women, when they are given HRT for the first time. That oestrogen has a direct effect on brain cells is well known, and these tests show that they can – so to speak – be wakened up again provided there is enough HRT reaching them in the blood stream.
>
> The women taking part in the trials were given regular brain scans. All the tests showed an increased level of activity amongst brain cells previously starved of oestrogen.

The patients were also given I.Q. tests before and after treatment and they all showed a significant improvement, which dropped back again when hormone replacement treatment was stopped", says the Report.

The American Study

In 1974 a survey was carried out by the local gynaecologist in Nashville, Tennessee, which drew on the medical records of the town's female inhabitants collected over a period of 30 years. He compared two groups of older women patients – one group who used HRT and the other who had not.

The number of breast cancers in HRT users was *half* that of the non-user group. Not only that, the incidence of *all forms* of cancer was lower in the user group as were other diseases of old age, including fractures caused by osteoporosis but also heart disease.

The survey indicated that the use of HRT not only delayed the onset of cancer by about 10 years, but it also slowed the general run-down in health. This was convincing proof that oestrogen is the body's first line of defence against infection, premature ageing and certain forms of cancer.

Evidence of the protective role of oestrogen throughout a woman's life grows stronger. It will not cure every ailment that comes with advancing years but it will certainly delay their onset, giving a better quality of life.

The British Study

The American study is not the only circumstantial evidence of the benefits which HRT can bring to older women. In her book on HRT, Wendy Cooper records similar observations made by a British doctor, John Maddison. He became convinced of the value of HRT when running a Geriatric Centre at Teddington, and carried out trials over a fifteen-year period.

> *"We observed the clinical state of some two thousand old people, taking regular checks for height, strength of hand-grip, mental ability and so on. Among the women half were given oestrogen and half were not. Those on oestrogen replacement showed no loss of height, while among the others there was up to two inches loss over the period due to osteoporosis. The ones on oestrogen also kept happier and more alert"*, he said.

These observations were not scientifically monitored but conducted over such a long period of time they are extremely valuable, not least because most of the elderly women using HRT managed to survive to the end of the trial!

These examples, albeit circumstantial, add to our general knowledge of the beneficial effects of HRT and provide powerful evidence of the long-term benefits of HRT. They certainly convince me that it is the best medical development for women since the contraceptive pill. So, let's go for it.

Old age is often idealised as a time to wind down and take life easy but a recent Report by the Commons Health Committee says that half a million elderly people suffer violence, bullying and theft at the hands of their 'carers' but are too frightened or too embarrassed to report their suffering. And, though it also takes place in 'care homes', it is much more common in their own homes – where even relatives lose patience with them because they are slow to understand or become doubly incontinent. Providing attendance allowance to enable elderly people to pay for help in their own homes doesn't solve the problem. But encouraging women at an earlier age to use HRT delays the ageing process and the need for permanent care in later life and a woman who retains her independence may also be able to offer support for her partner with a minimum of additional care.

The problem of what to do about an ageing population becomes more urgent when the government says that we will have to keep working until we are 70 without giving a thought as to whether people will be physically able to do so. Without HRT it will be impossible for most women of 70 to remain in employment - their health won't allow it – because older women are plagued with osteoporosis, strokes and a loss of mental ability. Sooner or later the government will have to come to terms with the fact that HRT is the only way guaranteed to prevent many of these problems and the astronomical costs that go with them.

What the rest of the world has to say about HRT

During my time as a Member of Parliament, and with the help of the excellent service of the House of Commons Library, I was able to monitor studies from around the world on the role of HRT. The message came through loud and clear: any link between the use of HRT and the risk of developing breast cancer is purely coincidental and that HRT is a good thing. But this type of survey is becoming out of date. It has been overtaken by genetic research into breast cancer which is taking place in universities all over the world.

Over is a small sample of the many surveys which have taken place over the last ten years.

The Division of Public Health Sciences, Cancer Research Center, Seattle. USA – July 1995.

Summary: "On the whole, oestrogen with progestogen HRT does not appear to be associated with an increased risk of breast cancer in middle-aged women. Compared with non-users of menopausal hormones, those who used oestrogen-progestogen HRT for eight or more years had, if anything, *a reduced risk of breast cancer on the whole"*

The Department of Obstetrics and Gynaecology, University of California at Irvine, College of Medicine, Orange, USA – November 1995.

Subject: Replacement therapy for breast cancer survivors.

Summary: "No significant adverse outcome was detected in cancer survivors receiving HRT".

Department of Family Medicine, Louisiana State University Medical Center, Shreveport, USA – July 1996.

Subject: The Review of literature following benefits from HRT studies.

Summary: "A *decrease* in urinary incontinence, *improvement* in emotional stability and relief from depression. Improved quality of life in patients with rheumatoid arthritis. Increased dermal and total skin thickness. Improved verbal skills and a *decrease* in the risk of colon cancer".

The Division of Epidemiology, University of Minnesota, Minneapolis, USA – December 1997.

Summary: "Among women with a family history of breast cancer, those who used HRT had a significantly *lower* risk from total mortality (death) than did women who had *never* used HRT. The age-adjusted mortality rate for women using HRT for at least five years is roughly *half* the rate seen in women who had never used HRT. These data suggest that HRT use in women with a family history of breast cancer is *not* associated with a significantly increased incidence of breast cancer but is associated with a significantly *reduced* total mortality rate".

Department of Radiology, University of Michigan Hospitals – September 1998.

Title: Breast Cancer in women who undergo screening mammography: Relationship of hormone replacement therapy to stage and detection method.

Result: "Among screened women who developed breast cancer, there were no significant differences in cancer stages or in the number of mammographically detected cancers between the HRT user group and the non-HRT group".

Chapter 16
MALE MID-LIFE CRISIS

*The Florida experience - Testosterone and men -
Is there a male menopause? - Genetic risks in
children of ageing fathers*

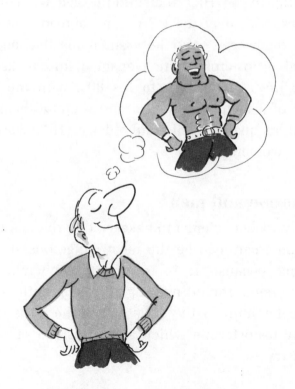

"The best thing to arouse a man with a mid-life crisis is a woman on HRT". Postcard seen in a telephone kiosk in Soho.

The Florida experience

"The State of Florida is one gigantic outdoor laboratory where millions of older women live life to the full, thanks to the benefits of HRT". Professor Robert Greenblatt, Professor of Endocrinology, Medical College of Georgia, USA.

I first met Professor Greenblatt – one of the great stars in the HRT firmament – at the International Congress On The Menopause held in Sorrento in 1987. Such was his reputation as an authority on HRT that middle-aged women flew into Georgia from all over the USA - and abroad – to have their implants renewed. And he assured me that he, too, took additional testosterone which enabled him to keep up his energetic life style. Then in his 80s, with the looks and charisma of a man half his age, testosterone therapy clearly enhanced his quality of life into old age. HRT works for men as well as women.

Testosterone and men

It's hardly rocket science to observe that the male hormone, testosterone, can also be the most dangerous substance on the planet because it is responsible for male violence towards women, including gang rapes and child abuse. The loutish behaviour on the streets after the pubs turn out is driven by testosterone which also fuels the sad and seedy sex industry.

From Arnold Schwarzenegger in the 'Terminator' and Tom Cruise in 'Top Gun', violent movies provide graphic illustration of how men view their assertiveness and they act as role models for impressionable young boys. The news about hormones in men is not all bad. They produce a certain amount of female hormone which acts as a civilising influence on their behaviour. The balance between these two powerful forces determines the degree of masculinity or femininity in both sexes.

Violent criminals are sometimes treated with progestogen, the female hormone, to bring their aggressive instincts under control. Some time in the future hormone adjustment may become a more widely accepted method of dealing with aggressive and dysfunctional male personalities.

Life expectancy for a man is about four years shorter than a woman but the ageing process in men has attracted much less interest. Between the ages of 30 and 70, men can lose a third of their bone mass but much less dramatically than in women. Still, it can lead to fractured hips, loss of height and a curved spine as testosterone declines. Prostate cancer is the commonest form of cancer in men and the female hormone progesterone is used to control it.

But the ageing male, or more specifically his reproductive system, has attracted less interest than older women.

Men claim to experience a mid-life crisis with a lack of concentration, tiredness and stress at work. Fear of failure at work coupled with a lacklustre home life may send them off in search of younger women in the hope that it will make them feel young again.

Is there a male menopause?

It used to be thought that reaching their half-century made men feel old but today's fiftysomethings claim to have a more enjoyable sex life than in their 30s and 40s – satisfaction triumphs over gratification! Menopause marks the end of a woman's fertility, so men do not go through a menopause. There is no clear break but most men seem to have psychological problems with growing old, particularly at work when they think they are being overtaken by younger men. Viagra came onto the market to cater for male impotence with NHS approval and is now prescribed without protest although it is known to increase the risk of a heart attack. And woe betide the government which tries to ban it after five years. Compare this with the constant sniping at HRT which is known to reduce the risk of heart attack in older women.

If middle-aged husbands rely on Viagra to keep them sexually active then

their middle aged wives will need HRT to keep up with them. It speaks volumes about the way in which society discriminates against older women. I doubt whether anyone within government has given this anomaly a thought.

The male 'menopause' could trigger heart disease as the level of testosterone falls. It is similar to changes affecting women over 50, who suffer rising levels of heart disease as they lose protection from their hormones. Vigorous sexual activity in older men can bring on a heart attack and, although it may not have been made public, I am aware of at least one Member of Parliament who died of a heart attack in his office whilst 'on the job'!

Genetic risks in children of ageing fathers

Men like to think that they can go on fathering children forever. It makes them feel young again and temporarily flatters their ego. Fatherhood in older men is always greeted with a mixture of surprise, curiosity and admiration. But sperm banks in the U.S.A. limit donors to men under 50 because of an increase in the number of children with Downs Syndrome born to fathers over 44 years of age. Research showed that 13% of sperm from older men had chromosome damage and *approximately one third of children born with Downs Syndrome were fathered by men over 40 years of age.* The risk is comparable to that of an older mother. Doctors were inclined to put this down to a drop in their testosterone levels, but there are no detailed studies to back this up.

Chapter 17
WHO CAN WE TRUST?

*Cherry picking time - Background to The Million
Women Study – The role of the Committee on Safety
of Medicines – The role of the cancer charities*

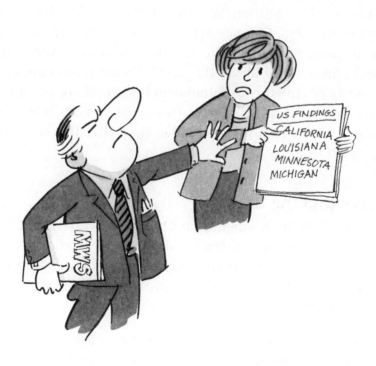

Dear Teresa,

"We would like to point out that a woman's chance of developing breast cancer is not limited to a strong family history of the disease. This study demonstrates that the risk of ten years use of combination HRT is comparable to having a mother and sister with breast cancer. There are many other risk factors too. These include: a woman's age the age a woman starts her period; the age a woman goes through menopause; the age of a woman's first pregnancy; having no children or few children; the contraceptive pill; being obese; drinking alcohol."

This letter was sent to me from Professor Valerie Beral, Director of The Million Women Study and Julietta Patnick, Director of NHS Cancer Screening Programmes, following critical comments made by me on the BBC. And funnily enough, Professor John Studd has much the same opinion but comes to a completely different conclusion. He points out that if you are looking for a cause there are many things in a woman's life you could blame other than HRT if you really set your mind to it.

Cherry picking time

A recent study by academics at Oxford University, published in the Journal of the American Medical Association, accused scientists of routinely cherry picking the result of surveys and failing to report 'inconvenient' findings in contravention of official guidelines on the reporting of research.

"In some cases the stated purpose of the survey is altered as it progresses so that acceptable findings are published, rather

than inconvenient results in order to satisfy the requirements of prestigious journals such as The Lancet, reducing them to the status of tabloid newspapers. Crucial information on survival rates is either downgraded in importance or omitted from the published report. Cherry picking of the results has serious implications for the reliability of recommendations made to the government or the NHS. There is a lot of pressure – and a lot of money at stake".

The background to The Million Women Study

In the opinion of many doctors and scientists the Million Women Study, was not conducted as a scientific study, although you would not have guessed it from the way it was hyped up to grab the headlines. It did *not* set out to find what causes breast cancer in middle-aged women but to discover whether there was a link between using HRT and the risk of developing the disease, ignoring the fact that the current scientific evidence leans towards breast cancer being largely hereditary.

The national average for breast cancer cases in older women is recorded as 45 per 1000. This study rose to 47 cases per 1000 of women using HRT – an extra two cases or 0.02% - well within the margin of error for a survey of this size and these extra cases could as easily be attributed to other causes. Furthermore, the women who took part in the survey were not selected at random from the population but from those already attending breast-screening centres which inevitably biased the result.

Recent research in Sweden found that rigorous screening over-diagnoses cancers and one in ten women are given unnecessary treatment for a cancer that would not have caused them any harm during their lifetime if they had not had treatment.

Even the British Menopause Society has been scathing in its views. They pointed out that the study population was not truly representative of the general population of women in the UK or of the treatment that women received during the six year study period. Compared with other clinical trials the risk was grossly overestimated.

This hasty decision was made by the same Committee which, in 1995, banned the contraceptive pill and had, subsequently, to withdraw its decision when, one year later, there was a massive increase in the demand for abortion. It was also the same committee that allowed Thalidomide to be prescribed to pregnant women *after* it had been banned in the USA.

Three years later, after the damage had been done, Professor Boyages, who led the MWS, backtracked on its original claims saying some women may have stopped the treatment *unnecessarily*. *"The risk of breast cancer from taking HRT is really quite small"*, he said. In other words, the Million Women Report gave misleading information which resulted in the health of millions of women being compromised because hormone replacement protects women from a number of diseases of old age. There was no attempt at the time on the part of the charity to correct the false impression given by the way the results of the survey were presented to the press.

When the first part of the Study was published in 1997, the country's leading scientific journal, The Lancet, was highly critical, *"Decisions have been driven by greed for publicity. The fundraising image of the cancer charity seem to have become their overriding priority causing confusion amongst women by selective reporting of the results"*. Unfortunately, the charity failed to take note of this criticism when they published the second part of the study in 2003.

The MWS fell far short of the rigorous standards which are demanded of medical research. It was a number-crunching exercise without the safeguards needed to give it scientific credibility. But scientific progress in the area of DNA will make these old-fashioned and gigantic studies obsolete by giving women - individually – precise information and peace of mind.

I also asked Douglas McWilliams, Chief Executive of Centre for Economics and Business Research, the country's leading authority in this field, for his opinion on the way in which this survey was conducted. This is what he had to say:

"In normal circumstances in large studies there is a degree of self-selection which may bias the results and I wonder how much correction for this has taken place. There appears to be a statistical correlation but this doesn't always mean cause and effect. As I understand it, there is no information about any medical process linking HRT and cancer and so the correlation is purely statistical".

Amongst other flaws were: no randomised trials, no control groups, and the fact that the charity conducting the survey had a vested interest in the result because it relies on public donations to support its activities. In my view the Study – spread over eight years and costing a small fortune – was not really worth the paper it was printed on. No doubt Professor Beral stands by her research and the conclusions drawn from them, and I imagine other doctors and scientists will support her. What cannot be doubted was that it heightened women's fear of developing breast cancer. The Report had the effect of frightening the life out of women who use HRT for sound medical reasons.

The MWS claimed they found an increase of two cases of breast cancer per *one thousand women* who took park in the survey. A similar study carried out by the Women's Health Initiative in the USA, came to the conclusion that the risk of breast cancer was even lower; seven cases *per ten thousand women* and no increase at all in the rate of heart disease. There have been 50 studies of HRT in the last 25 years, some of them falling well below the high standards of epidemiological proof required for evidence-based medicine. If these results are the worst they can come up with then we have nothing to be afraid of by using HRT. On the contrary, compared with the many benefits, it is the best thing for women since sliced bread!

The role of the Committee On Safety Of Medicines

The cancer charities are not the only ones to blame for this disaster. The government's way of dealing with health care is to create an army of bureaucrats producing a thicket of red tape which comes between the patient and the practitioners. What would the Ten Commandments have looked like if they had been run through the Committee on Safety of Medicines?

Advisory committees made up of nominees from industry and the professions – the great and the good - meet occasionally to consider and recommend to the government whether action should be taken on Reports, such as the MWS. The remit of this Committee is to "monitor the safety of marketed medicines and ensure that they meet acceptable standards of safety and efficacy".

Since most of the individuals serving on these committees have full-time jobs elsewhere, their decisions largely depend on recommendations made by 'working groups', whose advice they usually rubber stamp. In the case of the decision taken to ban HRT, Professor Beral who directed the Study for Cancer Research UK, also served as a member of the working group.

These committees do make mistakes – as in the case of the contraceptive pill - but, unlike Members of Parliament, they are not answerable to the public. The last thing they appear to think about is the effect their decisions have on the general public. The only way for a committee member to register disagreement is to resign, as did Professor Purdie because he knew how damaging the decision would be to women for whom HRT was essential in the prevention of osteoporosis.

The role of the cancer charities

Cancer charities rely heavily on public donations which are inevitably stimulated by scare stories in the Press. There are over 600 cancer charities in the UK; eighty of them breast cancer charities, all fishing in the same pond for funds. FM Radio recently carried an advertisement offering fundraisers for breast cancer the opportunity to earn £60,000 a year in commission, an insight into the amount of money to be made.

Not all charities are properly run. For example, in 1993 the Charity Commission had to appoint a Receiver to take over the running of a breast cancer charity in Scotland after concerns about serious mismanagement and complaints about the charity's fundraising methods. Only ten per cent of its multi-million pound income was spent on charitable work. The other 90% went on administration and fundraising expenses. These included £5 million paid to commercial fundraisers, two of whose employees were also charity trustees. This is not an isolated case.

The big players are multi-million pound organisations that rely on publicity to attract donations and legacies from the public, as well as tax breaks from the government. Not forgetting lottery funds. Parliament is currently debating new legislation to tighten regulations to ensure that charities stick to their proper role of benefiting the public at large. And then you will be able to know how much of the pound you put in the collecting box or the money you donate through your credit card actually helps the cause. In my opinion, breast cancer and other cancer charities don't deserve another penny until these reforms come into effect and they are forced to act responsibly.

Chapter 18
THE POLITICS OF HRT

'Braine' Storming – Contacting your MP – Time for the tea trolley – The free market to the rescue – Modern-day Suffragettes - Reversing the decision

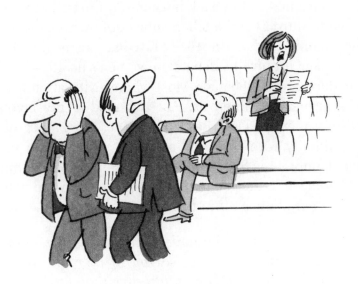

In 1987, when I was elected to Parliament, top of my list of priorities were two goals to improve life for women. One was Sunday Trading to save working women from tearing round the shops on a Saturday morning before they closed at lunchtime and the other was to put HRT on the map which I knew from personal experience could transform the lives of older women like myself.

My hope was to see a menopause clinic in every town and city and my election to Parliament gave me another opportunity to put HRT on the map by speaking on the subject in parliamentary debates.

'Braine' storming

The House of Commons is an overwhelmingly male, indeed chauvinistic, institution. Women's issues were, wherever possible, consigned to the back burner. So I regarded it as my big chance to introduce the taboo subject of menopause in the debating chamber when in 1987, Edwina Currie, the junior health minister, arranged a debate on women's health – the first time it had ever been debated. Most women MPs attended and a sprinkling of men joined us. As I warmed to my favourite subject - the menopause - Bernard Braine, the Father of the House, suddenly rose from his seat and stormed out of the debating chamber, his head bent forward muttering to himself. Bernard belonged to the generation when even married couples never took their clothes off in front of each other.

As I left the chamber at the end of the debate the doorman stopped me. *"What were you saying in there to upset Sir Bernard? He went past here muttering that he had never dreamt that he would hear such matters discussed in the Chamber"*, he asked.

Sir Bernard's reaction was fairly typical of the attitude that prevailed in society towards the subject menopause. And I suspect this feeling still lingers in Whitehall where NHS priorities are still decided by men and where older women are undervalued and under represented. I can guarantee that a debate on prostate cancer would be packed out.

Politicians are selective in the advice they choose to take. Professor Halligan, the Deputy Chief Medical Officer for the NHS, said *"HRT provided enormous benefits for women and far outweighed any potential risk"*. And Professor Purdie, one of the world's leading authorities on osteoporosis, condemned the Million Women Report and resigned from the government committee which had banned it.

"I believe GPs should retain the option to use HRT for women in their early 50s. HRT is effective, reliable and safe in preventing osteoporosis", he said.

If ever there was an open and shut case for reform this is it. The ban on HRT prescriptions must go, ASAP!

Contacting your MP

Members of Parliament are bombarded with the pleas of pressure groups to take on board their concerns – and pump public money into them. But if enough individual voters write to their MP on a particular subject they, too, can have an impact because each letter or phone call represents a potential vote. So let your MP know what you think about the shabby way menopausal women on HRT have been treated by the NHS. HRT, which has been used for decades by millions of women in other countries, guarantees you good health into old age and, given the government's concern about the prospect of an ageing population, this is a golden opportunity for them to do something about it. How else are women supposed to keep working until they are seventy – or longer - to avoid becoming a burden on the state?

You can contact your MP by writing to the House of Commons, London SW1A 0AA, or look up the local office in the telephone directory and pay them a visit at their 'surgery' and give them a piece of your mind! If a million or more women voters could be persuaded to take this course of action the NHS will be handing out HRT in gift-wrapped packages!

The opinion of Professor John Studd, a leading authority on HRT, is worth repeating:

> *"In the 50-59 year-old age group women using oestrogen-only therapy showed a decrease in cancer of 24%. The overall risk was no greater than the influence of being over-weight, drinking a little wine, having a late menopause or a late first pregnancy. HRT should not be withheld from post-menopausal women, since there is no evidence that the small amount of oestrogen in HRT increases their risk of breast cancer while added progestogen significantly reduces risk".*

Time for the tea trolley

Much of the tragedy and discomfort of old age is hidden from us. M.Ps regularly visit care homes in their constituency and however kindly the staff or comfortable the surroundings, the 'residents' seemed unaware of what is going on in the world around them or even recognise close members of their family. They doze all day until the tea trolley comes round. HRT means you can still go to the toilet on your own into your 80s.

The government is now warning us that we will all have to work five or ten years longer before we can draw our State pension, by which time most people are contemplating a move into sheltered housing. The numbers of us living into our 80s - and beyond - will double within 30 years. Today's 50 year-olds will have to work until their 70s in order to have enough to live on in retirement. But women, at least, can avoid the onset of dependency by taking HRT.

Most people are unaware of the extent of the problem that already exists in accommodating elderly people who are no longer able to look after themselves, much less work for their living. There are 600,000 people in the UK suffering from Alzheimer's but the government's 'rationing body' NICE (National Institute for Health and Clinical Excellence) is planning to withdraw drugs for this disease on the grounds of cost. This will leave patients without medication that has proved to be effective in slowing down the disease. If the government continues to withdraw funding for treatments that help us to live independently as we grow older it is no wonder that more and more people will have to be looked after in care homes.

The free market to the rescue

The UK government is making tentative moves to allow pharmacists a greater degree of freedom to dispense medicines which could, and should, include HRT. After all, HRT is not a drug – it simply replaces the body's natural hormones which disappear when menopause begins. HRT is not expensive. A month's supply can cost less than the current NHS charge. Pharmacists in your local chemist shop are perfectly capable of providing women with all the advice they need. This process would be speeded up if women in considerable numbers would write to their MP to demand that the serious consequences of the menopause are treated seriously because prevention is better than cure.

In almost every field - other than medicine - competition in the market place provides consumers with a variety of informed opinion and choice. But, when it comes to HRT women are kept in the dark on the relative merits of different products. And, in any case, they are unable to obtain them without the 'permission' of a third party – their GP - who is tempted to restrict the availability of popular products recommended for long term use in order to control the costs. Whilst in Parliament I monitored the increase in spending on HRT - a mark of its growing popularity. But in political terms, any treatment which involves increased expenditure is viewed with a jaundiced eye and ways to restrict its use are always in the forefront of the minds of the people who run the Health Service. In the case of HRT taking it off prescription would solve the problem then women can make up their own minds.

Despite the impression given by the breast cancer charities and the Press - there are no medical reasons for restricting the use of HRT. We have developed a decision-making process within politics which relies on the advice of committees rather than customer preference which is bound to result in cock-ups. The CSM is prone to cock-ups by banning first the contraceptive pill and then HRT.

The free market is like water – it finds its own level. It strives to give the customer what s/he wants while politicians seek to impose their often misguided opinions.

Modern-day Suffragettes

Two million women who have been refused HRT could have enormous political clout – if only they realised it. Properly organised they could put an end to the constant carping about HRT simply by contacting their MPs and demanding the reversal of this outrageous attack on their health. But organising women into a political lobby group is like trying to nail jelly to a wall.

The Women's Institute is persuaded that there is something 'not quite nice' about resisting the ravages of old age. And Age Concern, which campaigns against cruelty in old people's homes, says not a word in support of HRT which would keep women out of care homes. Private medical insurance excludes HRT treatment from their policies – preferring to let the NHS foot the bill – knowing full well that major surgery may be needed at a later date to repair the results of untreated menopause – thus cutting off their nose to spite their face.

By limiting long-term use of HRT the government is storing up hugely expensive medical problems for the future, despite the fact that it is easy, effective and inexpensive to prevent them. As a result, orthopaedic wards will continue to be filled with elderly women patients recovering from fractures which could have been avoided. To say nothing of the other indignities of old age.

Government health policy is built around crisis management rather than preventative medicine, of which HRT is probably the worst example of sex discrimination in the NHS. There's no quibbling about providing Viagra prescriptions for middle-aged men but hormone replacement for women is cut off after five years and women are denied the right to buy it over the counter. But, unless women are prepared to make a fuss - the squeaky wheel gets the most grease - these inequalities will continue and women will always be left at the end of the queue.

Reversing the decision

The government decision to limit access to HRT to a five-year period will have profound long-term medical repercussions. The health and well being of two million women is at stake. Irreversible physical damage in the form of osteoporosis will return if access is limited to five years and is already taking place where HRT treatment has been discontinued. The cost of treating women who will develop this disease will mushroom in years to come. The problem with politicians is their myopia - they can't see beyond the next election – five years ahead.

The currency of politics is votes and the threat of losing the votes of two million women on HRT at the next election is one of the few constraints which might actually change the government's mind. I hope that this book will add to their discomfort by increasing pressure on them to reverse this wholly unacceptable interference in a woman's choice. HRT – which is only used by older women – has so many benefits that the sooner we get the message across the better. Consultant gynaecologists view the Million Women Study with scorn. The ban on HRT was a political and financial decision. It is not medically valid and must be reversed.

Chapter 19
YOUR QUESTIONS ANSWERED

"The quality of your life depends on the questions you ask." Here are some of the questions that I get asked from time to time.

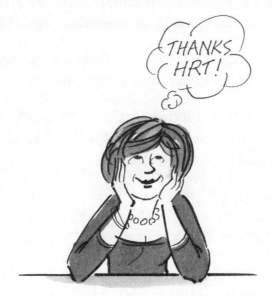

<u>Late Pregnancy</u> - Just when you think your periods are over and you have given up taking precautions or the Pill you could find yourself pregnant all over again. Ovaries sometimes have a late fling and produce an egg. If you decide to go through with the pregnancy then you must stop taking HRT at once.

<u>Deep Vein Thrombosis</u> - (blood clots in the legs) there is no evidence linking it to HRT but it has been suggested that it is linked to use of the Pill.

<u>Leg Cramps</u> – are thought to be linked to high levels of female hormones in the blood stream. If cramps are very bad or very frequent try leaving off your HRT for a couple of days and consult your GP if it occurs regularly. Or try Crampex tablets which can be bought over the counter.

<u>Varicose Veins</u> – are inherited from either side of your family. There is no known connection between them and HRT.

<u>Heavy Smoking</u> – Can contribute to heart attacks while HRT reduces the risk of both heart attacks and strokes.

<u>Breast cancer</u> – and other forms of cancer - runs in families and there is no evidence that HRT increases the risk. Check your family history and have a DNA test.

<u>Gallstones and Liver Problems</u> – can be aggravated if HRT is taken by mouth. Women with these problems must use some other form of HRT such as a skin patch or implant.

<u>Fibroids</u> – are funny little outgrowths of the skin which sometimes appear in odd places but have nothing to do with HRT. They are usually harmless and can easily be removed.

<u>Will I get fat?</u> – Only if you eat too much. Menopause can make you feel miserable and resort to 'comfort' eating. As you get older you don't need as much food.

<u>When should I start using HRT?</u> – When you get irregular periods, hot flushes, night sweats, etc., etc. See the chapter on Menopause Symptoms.

<u>How long must I take HRT?</u> – As long as you want to. Of course, you can stop it whenever you like but you risk the problems returning. I've used HRT for 30 years and I'm fit as a fiddle and I have arranged for a packet to be placed in my coffin, just in case!

<u>What are the catches?</u> – If you still have your womb you will get a sort of mock period each month. Doctors call it a "withdrawal bleed". Some women don't mind this. It makes them feel they are still young. At first you may get tender breasts, feel hungry, or experience cramps in your calves. But this will go away once the dose is right. In any case, this is a small price to pay for the many benefits which are terrific.

<u>Will HRT help to stop my bones becoming brittle?</u> – Yes. Medical research shows that a lack of the 'O' hormone is the main cause of bone decay. By the time you reach 70 you have a one in four chance of having a major bone fracture and some women will die from it.

<u>Does calcium help prevent bone decay?</u> – No matter how much calcium you consume, your body cannot use it to protect your bones without the presence of sufficient 'O' hormone. The two go hand in hand.

Is HRT suitable for everyone? – No treatment ever is. There are several ways of taking HRT and your GP will need to try out various methods in order to find one which suits you. But if your GP turns you down you can go private or turn to the Internet.

SUMMARY

'The change' may be a natural event which all women must face. But it is also a form of deficiency disease, no different in principle from diabetes which is caused when the body can no longer make the hormone, insulin. Replacing missing hormones is a well-established medical practice. Now it can be done for the menopause. It's true that past generations of women have had to put up with it because there was nothing to be done.

Hormone replacement is preventive medicine at its best. It's up to you to decide whether you want to take it. But don't let anyone else make the decision for you.

APPENDIX I

Survey of the literature on the biology of breast cancer by Dr. Amineh Abu Zayyad, PhD

Much effort has been put into understanding the genetics of predisposition to breast cancer as well as identifying factors involved in tumor progression and cancer prognosis (Sauer M.K.; 2002). Biological characteristics such as expression levels, protein stability and phosphorylation as well as the biological roles of breast cancer (BRCA) proteins in DNA repair and transcription have led to the identification of other proteins involved in breast cancer. Intensive research in an effort to prevent and find treatment for cancer has revealed that damage to some types of genes, for example the Ras genes, create oncogenes which encode proteins which lead to the uncontrolled proliferation characteristic of cancer cells ((Nalca A. *et al*, 1999; Treeck 0. *et al*;2003). Evidence pointing to the role of Rho-dependent pathways and their interaction with oncogenic Ras in contributing to 131 cell cycle abnormalities which characterize human breast cancer has been intensively studied, (Ridley &J.; 2004, Welsh; 2004, Wu M. *et al*; 2004). It is believed that Rho family of GTPases plays a large role in cell proliferation, invasion and metastasis.

Somatic changes in the genome of breast cancer cells include amplifications, deletions and gene mutations. Several chromosome regions harboring oncogenes are found amplified in breast tumors. For example a decade of studies of the long arm of chromosome 20 (20q) has been observed in a wide variety of cancers, one of them is breast cancer. This suggests that a gene or genes encoded on 20q play important roles in contributing to the cancer proliferation when over expressed (Hodgson J.G. *et al*; 2003). Gene discovery efforts have revealed a number of interesting candidate genes on chromosome 20 that may contribute to oncogenIc progression and proliferation of cancer cells (Ethier SP., 2003). On the other hand some studies show that the CTCF gene may be involved in tumor initiation or proliferation in individual cases of invasive ductal breast carcinomas (Aulmann S. et al; 2003, XL Z. *et al.*; 2004, Tonin PN. 2000).

Breast Cancer Genes

The most well documented and intensely studied genes are BRCAI and BRAC2, which are tumor suppressor genes (anti-Oncogenes), which are normally involved in cell growth regulation. They inhibit cell proliferation, which is crucial for normal cell development and differentiation. Germ-line mutations in those tumors predispose women and men to breast cancer (Coughlin 5.5. era); I999, Dalpe R. *et al*; 2003, Gayther SA *et al*; 1998, Rhan p., 1996, Pasca A. *et al*; Wooster R. *et al*; 1995, 2002, Welcsh P.L. *et al*; 2001, Wooster R. *et al*; 1995; Aretini *et al*, 2003, King *et al.*, 2003). These genes can be passed from parent to child, increasing a lifetime risk of developing cancer in that child.

There is a very high risk of developing breast cancer in women carrying these mutated genes. Men carrying the BRCAI have no risk of developing breast cancer, but those carrying the BRCA2 genes have a very high risk of developing breast cancer or prostate cancer (Aretini P. *et al*; 2003, Gayther S.A.; 2000, Anderson W.F. *et al*; 2004; Pasca A. *et al*; 2002). So a man with the mutated BRCA2 gene is just as likely to pass this gene on to his children as a woman with this mutated gene. There is a

90% chance of developing breast cancer for a person carrying these mutated genes. Some studies have noted that male breast cancer is more likely to develop later in life (postmenopausal, Anderson WE. *et al*; 2004).

Progress in determining the function of BRCAI and BRCA2 suggests that they are involved in two fundamental cellular processes: DNA damage repair and transcriptional regulation, (lngvarsson S.; 1999, Somasundaram K. *et al*; 1997). For example studies on lymphoblastoid cell lines using a micronucleus test technique, have given another strong indication that women carrying BRCAI mutation develop breast cancer (Trenz K. *et al*; 2003).

BRCA1

BRCA1 was identified in 1990 and was isolated in chromosome 17 (17q) in 1994. Chromosome 17 is one of the 23 pairs of chromosomes found in most human cells. An altered BRCAI has been linked to the development of breast and ovarian cancer. However preliminary studies have shown that testing positive for an altered BRCAI gene does not necessarily mean a woman will develop breast cancer. At least 15% of the women who carry the altered gene will never develop the disease. Scientists have no way yet of knowing which women fall into that category. In addition, because BRCA1 alterations occur in many different regions scattered throughout the gene. Developing an accurate test is difficult to do.

BRCA2

BRCA2 was isolated on chromosome 13 (13q) in 1995. lnheriting a damaged version of the gene gives women a high risk of developing breast and ovarian cancer, and men of developing breast and prostate cancer. BRCA2 is now allowed to be used free for research in Europe (Cancer Research U K).

Some other Reported breast cancer genes

The risk of breast cancer is probably influenced by other unidentified genes with individual risk that is much smaller than the effect of the BRACI and BRCA2 whose contribution is large. Many molecular pathways, scientists believe, lead to breast cancer. Many reported oncogenes were found and reported in literature (Brody L. *et al*; 1998. Ormiston W 1995. Kinzler et a!; 1997. Marx J. I997. Rivera-Varas V. 1998. Sinclair U.S. *et al:* 2003; Setiawan VW: 2004). Some of these genes were summarized as follows:

P53

Protein 53 is a tumour suppressor gene, which plays a major role in cell growth. It suppresses cells from growth; if it is damaged or altered it loses its ability to block cell growth. Changes to the gene result in an increased risk of cancer-BRCAI has been reported to be expressed in a cell cycle-dependent manner; possesses transcriptional activity; associated with several proteins, including the p53; and play an integral role in certain types of DNA repair: Studies have shown that high density DNA array screening identified several genes affected by BRCAI expression in p53 in an independent manner, including DNA damage response genes and genes involved in cell cycle (MacLachlan T.K., et aI: 2000; Wojapeyee N., and Somasundaram K. 2003). This means that BRACI has the potential to modulate the expression of genes and function of proteins involved in the cell cycle control and DNA damage response pathways.

ATM

The gene, ataxia telangiectasia mutated (ATM) is a recessive gene found on chromosome 1, which may be involved in many cancers, including breast cancer. Its normal role is to control cell division and when damaged or altered it causes cancer (Scott S.S. *et al*; 1990: Shigeta T. *et al* 1999).

Known as the Cowden disease gene, an altered form of this gene is linked to both breast and prostate cancers.

CYR6l

Is a secreted, cysteine-rich, heparin binding protein that promotes endothelial cell adhesion, migration, and neo-vascularzation. Analysis of this gene revealed that Cyr6l was expressed highly in the invasive breast cancer cell lines MDA-MB-231, and MDA-MB-157; very low levels were found in the less tumorigenic MCF-7 and BT-20 breast cancer cells and barely expressed in the normal breast cells (MCF-12A 9Xie D. *et al*; 2001).

Some Reported Examples of Familial Breast Cancer

The following are a few examples of reported data from studies on familial breast cancer. There are many other examples that are reported in the literature.

Australian Women

In a study carried out in Australia, it has been found that the lifetime risk of developing breast cancer is 8.6% (1 in 12) for the general population, and it is 7.8% (1 in 13) for those without a family history. Women with one relative affected have lifetime risk of I in 6-8 and those with two relatives affected have lifetime risk of 1 in 4-6 (Tylor R. *et al.*; 2000). This study is another indication that women with family history of the disease are at a higher risk.

Ashkinazi Jewish population

The isolation of BRCA1 and BRCA2 genes allowed doctors and researchers to conduct methods and ways for screening in families with history of developing the disease. In a study of familial multiple cases of breast and ovarian cancer in Ashkinazi Jewish families for possible alterations in BRCA1 and BRCA2 has found a single BRCA1 mutation called l85delAG is commonly seen in breast and ovarian cancers (Genetic & IVF: Online, Struewing JP. *et al*; 1995; Struewing JP. *et al*, 1997). This genetic alteration has been estimated to account for 20% of cases of breast cancer and 39% of ovarian cancer in the Ashkinazi women before age 50. In addition, two other BRCA2 mutations seem to be over-represented in the Ashkinazi Jewish population. Although other types of mutations in BRCAI and BRCA2 do exist in the general population, these mutated types that were associated with the Ashkinazi families were only found in the Ashkinazis, and not in the general population. Other studies found that women carrying the mutant form of BRCAI may have up to 85% risk of developing breast cancer and a 44% risk of developing ovarian cancer in their lifetime. This compares to an overall 12% risk of breast cancer and 1% of ovarian cancer in the whole generation (Coughlin S.S. et al; 1999, Fergus K. et al; 2000, Struewing JP. *et al*, 1995; Steinberg K.K *et al*; 1998,). In addition to breast and ovarian cancers in women, prostate and breast cancer has been reported in Ashkinazi men due to the inherited BRCAI and BRCA2 genes (Giusti R.M. *et al*; 2003; Kirchhoff T. *et al*, 2004; Struewing J.P. *et al*, 1999).

African American

Another example of familial breast cancer was reported by a four-generation family survivor. Three generations were diagnosed with breast cancer but the fourth generation, who was diagnosed with breast cancer at age 32, survived the disease after two separate mastectomies (Brown Z.K., 2000).

Czech Republic

A complete coding sequence analysis of both BRCA1 and BRCA2 was carried out on 197 patients from high-risk families and 53 patients with sporadic breast/ovarian cancer. It has been found that 59 mutations (16 different) in BRCAI and 29 mutations (17 different) in BRCA2 were identified in unrelated breast/ovarian index cases. Five mutations in both BRCA1 and BRCA2 were represented, a total of 56.8% of all detected mutations. A broad spectrum of other mutations were detected including another four novel mutations (Foretova L. *et al.*, 2004). In summary, this study concluded that the harmful mutations were in 40.6% of 197 high-risk families and 37.5% in 16 patients with sporadic breast cancer.

Genetic testing, Counseling and (Hope for Treatment & Prevention)

Genetic testing might be controversial, but I believe genetic counseling and testing is a way to understand the nature of the disease, severity, and prognosis and whether or not there is an effective treatment. Genetic testing should be offered for women with a strong family history of breast cancer. If the woman is carrying the mutated gene she can be offered strict regular breast screening tests, or even the removal of her ovaries, and monitoring and avoid the pain and the severity of the disease. It is also recommended that women with high risk should follow a healthy diet and lifestyle (Bodd T.L. *et al* 2003, Pearson, 2003; Kenen *et al*; 2003).

There is no certain way of preventing breast cancer, but scientists are hoping that they can use genes to replace the defective ones, or to develop drugs to strengthen the defective DNA repair pathway (Ponder B. A. J., 1997; Russo *et al.*, 2003).

There are hopes for using a combined treatment consisting of anti-estrogen and vitamin D analogs. Metastatic tumors normally progress after a period of response to treatment and an endocrine treatment is needed, but an estrogen-dependent growth develops. It had been found that the growth of breast cancer cells is sensitive to the anti-estrogens combined with vitamin D analogues and inhibits their growth. (Christensen G.L. *et al*, 2004, Swami S. *et al*, 2003).

Aspartic Protease Gene (ALP56) recently identified as Cathepsin D [a lysosomal aspartic protease produced in human breast cancer cell lines has mitogenic activity in breast cancer] may be a useful target in the treatments of breast cancer (Kondoh K.; 2003).

BRCA1 & BRCA2

Soon after the discovery and cloning of the BRCAI and BRCA2 mutations, companies and research laboratories began offering genetic testing for individuals interested in knowing whether they are carrying these mutations (Chappuis P. *et al*; 2001, Jakubowska A. *et al*; 2003, Renwick A.A. *et al*; 2000, Wonderlick *et al.* 1997); however, genetic testing of BRCAI and BRCA2 is controversial. Tests may not provide useful information; scientists cannot predict who will get breast cancer or how severe its manifestations might become.

ATM

Although scientists do not know why an altered ATM gene causes cancer, 1% of the Americans carry at least one copy of the defective gene. By examining the role of the altered genes, scientists are hoping to shed some light on what makes cells live, grow and die. ATM may also identify those individuals who are sensitive to radiation.

P65

The altered form of P65 is linked to the overproduction of certain hormones that may help in developing breast and prostate cancer. The new blood test, called the tumor blood marker, may allow doctors to monitor a patient's response to cancer treatment. The level of P65 protein marker in the blood decreases as tumors are destroyed during cancer therapy.

P53

Almost 50% of all human cancer cells contain a P53 mutation. These cancers are very aggressive and fatal. Since it is so important for normal cell growth, scientists are continuing to research for ways to diagnose, prevent, and treat cancers associated with P53 (Lai H. *et al*; 2004).

Other hopes in the treatment and prevention of Breast Cancer

Integrins as mediators of the metastasis of breast cancer

The most dangerous stage in breast cancer is the spread of the tumor to other parts of the body (metastasis). Tumor cells need adhesion molecules to migrate to other regions of the body. If the activity of such adhesion molecules could be inhibited, then the metastasis of cancer could be slowed down and perhaps result in the elimination of the tumor. These adhesion molecules are called *integrins*; they are a large group of transmembrane glycoproteins that bind to adhesive macromolecules in extracellular matrices and on cell surfaces. They are adhesive receptors and make a dominant process of cell-cell and cell-substratum adhesion (Abu-Zayyad A. PhD, 1997; Hynes, 1992; Turner *et al,* 1991). Integrins had been linked to diverse fields of haematology, neurobiology, thrombosis, inflammation, AIDS, development and biology of cancer. Decades of research of integrins and their role in cancer have concluded that they play a key role in cancer; they are mediators of the metastasis and breast cancer. The progression of breast cancer is now known as a result of a series of genetic alteration, and the hypothesis is that the integrin adhesion molecules signal to the cell to start the genetic alteration which leads to the development and the progression of cancer.

Much research has been carried out to understand this process and how to inhibit and eliminate the development of breast cancer, ovarian and other cancers. For example the essential role of the integrin receptor avb3 in metastasis has been studied and it has been shown that this is essential in invasion and metastasis. It has been reported that some polymorphic genetic variation of integrins expressed in platelets and epithelial breast cells could modify the risk of the biological aggressiveness of breast cancer (Ayala A. *et al* 2003, Bojesen S.T. *et al*; 2003, Qianren J. *et al*; 2004). In some cases an adhesion molecule (fibronectin) has been reported to provide a survival protection to breast cancer cells *in vitro*: a suggestion for a promising therapy in the near future (Newton S.A. *et al*; 1995, Wieder R. *et al* 2003).

APPENDIX II

Menopause Clinics

Clinics in the South East

Miss Joan Pitkin
Consultant Obstetrician & Gynaecologist
Northwick Park Hospital
Watford Road
Harrow
Middlesex HA1 3UJ

Professor John Studd
The Lister Hospital (Private)
Chelsea Bridge Road
London SW1W 8RH

PMS & Menopause Clinic
120 Harley Street
London W1N 1AG

Professor Janice Rhymer
Guy's Nuffield House
Guy's Hospital
London SE1 1YR

Guy's and St Thomas Menopause Clinic
McNair Centre
Thomas Guy House
Guy's Hospital
London SE1 lYR

Menopause Clinic
Department of Gynaecology
3rd Floor

Golden Jubilee Wing
King's College Hospital,
Denmark Hill
London SE5 9RS

Clinics in East Anglia

Menopause Clinic
Colchester General Hospital
Constable Wing
Turner Road
Colchester
Essex CO4 5LJ

Caroline Marfleet
Isis Fertility Centre
Newcomen Way
Severalls Business Park
Colchester
Essex CO4 9YA

Clinics in the South West

Poole Menopause Centre
St Mary's Gynaecology Unit
Poole Hospital
Longfleet Road
Poole BH15 2JB

Clinics in the Midlands

Mr Michael P Cust
Derby Nuffield Hospital
Rykneld Road
Derby DE23 4SN

Menopause Clinic
Derby City General Hospital
Uttoxeter Road
Derby DE22 3NE

Menopause Clinic
University Hospital of North Staffordshire
Newcastle Road
Stoke on Trent
Staffordshire ST4 6QG

Professor P M S O'Brien
Nuffield Hospital
Clayton Road
Newcastle Under Lyme
Staffs ST5 4DB

David Sturdee
Menopause Clinic
Department of Women's Health
Solihull Hospital
Lode Lane
Solihull B91 2JL

David Sturdee
BUPA Parkway Hospital
Damson Parkway
Solihull B91 2PP

Clinics in Northern England

Menopause Clinic
Nuffield Hospital Leeds
2 Leighton Street
Leeds LS1 3EB

Menopause Clinic
Leeds General Infirmary
Gynaecology Outpatients
Clarendon Wing
General Infirmary
Belmont Grove
Leeds LS2 9NS

Menopause Clinic
Pinderfields General Hospital
Gynaecology Outpatients
Aberford Road
Wakefield WF1 4DG

Menopause Clinic
St James' University Hospital
Chancellor Wing
Beckett Street
Leeds LS9 7TG

Tony Mander
Lancaster House
174 Chamber Road
Oldham
Lancashire OL8 4BU

Clinics in Scotland

Menopause Clinic
Dumfries and Galloway Royal Infirmary
Bankend Road
Dumfries DG1 4AT

ALSO BY TERESA GORMAN

Slow to Hire, Quick to Fire

Worried to Death

Qualgos Slugs and Paranoid Aardvarks

Business Still Burdened

The Enterprise Culture

The Amarant Book of Hormone Replacement Therapy

Chickengate

The Bastards

A Parliament for England

No, Prime Minister!